Nature's Gateway

To Health

By

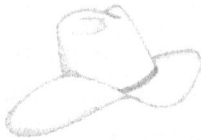

George *Walters*

To Be Able To Heal Oneself Naturally
Is The Greatest Gift Of All

Disclaimer

The information in this book is provided for general informational purposes only. It is not intended to replace, substitute for, or supersede professional medical advice, diagnosis, or treatment. Laws and regulations regarding natural health products vary by province and country.

Because we have no knowledge of your personal health history or any pre-existing conditions you may have, it is strongly recommended that you consult with a licensed physician or qualified medical practitioner before using or practicing any of the methods, foods, herbs, or natural substances described in this book. This is especially important if you are pregnant, nursing, taking prescription medications, or have known allergies or sensitivities.

This book is not meant to diagnose or treat any medical condition. For diagnosis or treatment of any medical problem, consult your own physician or a qualified health professional.

The author, publisher, sellers, distributors, and bookstores shall not be held liable under any circumstances, including but not limited to negligence, for any special, incidental, or consequential damages arising from the use of, or the inability to use, the information presented in this book.

Be aware that certain foods, herbs, and natural substances can cause serious allergic reactions or harmful side effects in some individuals. Some people have died from allergic reactions to plants and foods that others use without any problem at all.

Everything discussed in this book carries potential risk. If you are seriously ill, that risk increases significantly. Proceed carefully, and always seek qualified medical guidance first.

This book is intended for informational purposes only and does not constitute medical advice under Canadian law or the laws of any other jurisdiction.

Published 2015

ISBN: 978-0-9809884-8-2

Also by George Walters

~~~

Books by George Walters
Illustrations by Ruth Walters

Life Stories and Reflections

One More Story
Moments in Time
Paths We Choose
Keep Turning Pages
Times Changin'

Natural Living

Join Me In The Garden

I would also like to take a moment to tell you about a new series.
Strange Occurrences
The Clay Moretti Files — Book One
Available now on Amazon. More books in the series coming soon.
George Walters

Illustration's

By

Ruth Walters

Ruth is a self-taught artist, her artistic talents easily draw the reader into this world of healing. She opens your mind to a more naturalistic way of being with Nature.

Her drawings of trees, herbs and plants in their natural state are brought forth so that they are easily recognized in their own habitat.

Her talents make for a magical blend which I am sure will inspire you to create and support a healthy way of life.

Praise For This Book

George and Ruth Walters are dear personal friends of mine. One of the many things we have in common is our shared interest in wellness and healing. For us, wellness or good health is the state brought forth by the combination of three things—good genes, good fortune and good health habits. One doesn't often think about the first two "goods" because there's not much a person can do to improve the odds if genetics and / or bad luck conspire to rob one's health.

On the bright side, good health habits can be adopted and practiced by everyone. They contribute to well-being and can often counterbalance the negative effects of things that are felt to be, beyond our direct control. We know about the importance to our health of good nutrition and daily exercise but practicing good personal hygiene, breathing clean air, drinking pure water, getting enough refreshing sleep, avoiding toxins, maintaining a positive attitude and having good relationships with family and friends are equally important.

Wellness is not my only medical interest. The study of various forms of healing is also my passion and (strange as it may seem) a hobby of sorts. I enjoy tracing the origins and history of Western medical practice from its inception in Ancient Greece and Rome up to the Middle Ages, into the renaissance era and through to modern times. Schools of natural medicine, osteopathy, surgery, physical medicine (chiropractic) and homeopathy to name just a few, have had many centuries of development and have all contributed to our understanding of "modern medicine". So too has the wisdom and learning of indigenous healers.

George and Ruth have written a book which discusses some natural treatments that have been used by traditional healers for centuries here in North America. In this regard, the book is a gem—a repository of knowledge from the field of natural medicine which is not only fascinating from a historical perspective but could serve as a valuable reference resource as well. The book is not intended to stand alone as a primer of self-treatment for Naturopathy. Anyone interested in using natural remedies should first seek a consultation from an expert in the field.

George and I have great respect for each other (as friends should). Naturally, the ideas and opinions expressed in the book are his own and there are things upon which we don't necessarily agree. He, for instance, has reservations about vaccines. I believe that on the whole, vaccines are good and have saved many millions of people on the planet from disability and untimely death.

Ultimately, one must decide for themselves on the best course of action to be taken and take responsibility for his or her own health.

That said, I have the deepest appreciation for the work that George and Ruth have put forth to complete this book.

I congratulate them on a task well done.

Graham L. Wood MD

Praise For This Book

The whole point of science is to find the truth, not based on opinion, but mere facts that we have confirmed, and gathered over the years. It is the only model that we have today which actually causes us to get better at it.

I agree the medical and pharmaceutical companies need work though, since money has an impact on how they invest. Luckily the universities that are doing research around the world actually care about the results and people.

Karl Walters

To My Readers

✧ ✧ ✧

In more than forty years of setting words to paper and over two thousand published stories written, not one of those years passed without my readers finding their way to me. Letters that came by post and emails that arrived in the quiet of the morning. Phone calls from people I had never met yet somehow knew. And yes, folks who took the time to drive out and knock on our door.

You came to tell me the stories meant something, and they helped, and they made you laugh or cry or remember someone you loved. I read every letter and I answered every call and I welcomed every one of you who came. There are no words enough to thank you properly so I will simply say this — You kept me writing.

George Walters

*This Book Is Dedicated
To*

*My Lovely Wife Ruth
And
My Sons Karl and Craig*

Acknowledgements

First and foremost, I would like to thank my wife Ruth for her love, encouragement, and unfailing support. She once again brought feeling, meaning, and life into view for all to see. There were many times I had all but given up on writing this book, only to be brought back by her voice of assurance.

I would also like to thank my sons, Karl and Craig, for their support and guidance. At times their views differed from mine, but their perspective was a valuable part of completing this book.

I thank my father, who taught me wit and the value of a dollar. His views on life will always remain with me.

Reg and Laura Potter, an elderly couple who took me in and raised me as their own when my parents couldn't, taught me what it means to be strong in both mind and spirit.

My friend Dr. Graham Wood and his wife Janette stood beside my wife and me in times of need, offering their support and advice freely, and most of all, their friendship.

Allan Lawry, for his kind words and article on cholesterol.

Bob Bartlett, for his poems—it was a difficult decision which one to include, as all were worthy.

Then there is Grey Wolf, my Native friend from years ago. His knowledge and teachings are woven throughout these pages. He played a great role in my upbringing, teaching me the importance of helping others, and myself. Every day, I miss his strength, wisdom, and gentle smile.

And finally, I thank you—my readers—who over the years have given me the encouragement to continue writing these books.

Table of Contents

Preface

Plants you have to remember do not heal everything. Sometimes we look to the earth or animals for help. Sometimes the power of touch.

I have come to the conclusion that even though a lot of these work quite well, how they work is still a mystery. I have also decided that I do not really need to know why.

I believe that we think too much and then in other instances I have found some don't think at all.

There are times I have found that I don't want to wait for things to start happening. That's when I have to step back and draw in the energy that is around me. In doing so I can wait.

Sometimes the shortest path isn't the best path, if I can just be patient and focused on the moment, I won.

Many times Grey Wolf was asked. What is the secret to staying young. His reply was; "Get the thoughts of getting old out of your mind." That is the real secret. You look and feel as old as you act.

One needs to laugh a lot, eat well, be in touch with the energy that surrounds you and most of all always have something to look forward to.

Also remember. Once you have used these Natural remedies and become well discontinue use. Listen to your body it will tell you when you have had enough.

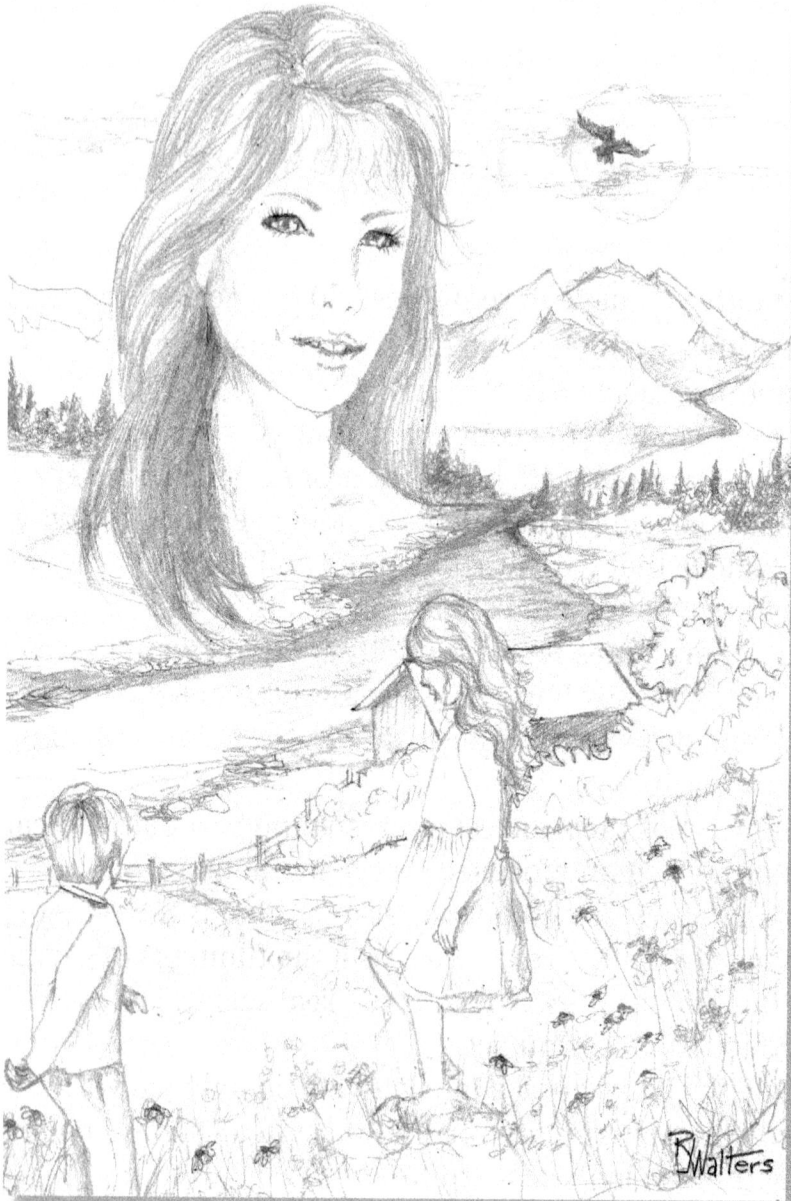

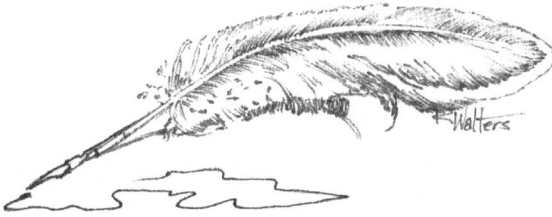

Natures Gateway To Health

I learned early in life that we are here to help one another. That thought along with many requests is how this book came into being.

One has to start at the beginning to grasp what Nature has to offer. Starting with the people who took the time using experimentation, hard work and even death sometimes, to bring together the actual abilities that plants and Nature have to offer.

This book is full of wisdom and knowledge, taken from the present along with the past.

Grey Wolf told me many times; there can be no healing without real or genuine love and kindness, for the person that needs healing.

He also said that our bodies are not all that we have. Our spirits live on after our body has perished, and a healthy spirit is just as important as a healthy body, if not more.

Starting out there weren't very many drugs available, other than what the Natives had. If only we had listened to what they had to offer and supported their way of life. In doing so, I feel that many of today's diseases and body ailments would not exist.

For myself growing up, I never heard of any pharmaceutical drugs to speak of, other than what was sold at our local hardware store. The owner would sell or trade a bit of laudanum to those that were in desperate need, most though

1

was handed out by the doctor of the town. And rightly so, as too much could cause more harm than good.

Today there are thousands of drug stores, almost one on every corner. Is that a good thing?

It's my opinion that things have gotten too complicated, and I believe that most minds have been swayed into thinking nature isn't helpful. It's a shame, as there is so much to learn when it comes to Nature.

I at one time almost headed off on roads that could have destroyed my life, only to be drawn back into reality.

"Reality," my friend Grey Wolf used to say, "is what is right in front of us, that most choose to ignore."

While I have Grey Wolf on my mind, let me introduce him to you. He was a great fellow, a Native American chap that lived in a small cottage by a creek on our property, many years ago. At the time I was around ten years of age, and he would be in his seventies. A man full of knowledge, from making flutes to treating humans and animals of all kinds, using only his homemade remedies, which came from Nature herself.

Walking into his cabin, one could see shelves of all kinds, stocked full of dried leaves, mushrooms, herbs, barks and much more. Most of my remedies I use today have come from his collection of recipes. Great man, and we will get back to him, and some of his treatments as these pages unfold.

But first, there are others that I have learned from, like my father, Earl Walters, a great man and so full of wisdom.

His remedies were mostly related to what was right in life, like living a healthful lifestyle and making the most out of each day. Hard work also played a good part in his life, but only to the extent of always having time to sit and chat with others if the need arose.

He also taught me the value of things in life, like what a fair price was for items of need and not be taken to the cleaners so to speak.

Another woman by the name of Laura might say she was my second Mother. Laura Potter, she knew more about helping folks in need and mending wounds than I could begin to tell you. She would never let anyone go without treatment, and if things came upon her she did not know, she would seek out those that could help.

Reg was her husband, another great fellow, who could mend a broken leg of a human or critter and make it feel good while doing it. Had a way about him that one could relax when near.

Then there was Nancy. Nancy was Reg and Laura's daughter. In her own way, she helped many a person using nothing more than kindness. Many days were spent chatting with her around the old wood stove, which in turn brought things back into their right perspective.

My Grandfather, now there was a man. Travelled throughout the USA and Canada surveying for different railways for most of his life, on horseback most of the time, working with Nature in the raw. I am in the process of writing a book on his life story which I am sure most will find quite entertaining.

He taught me much in life which I will share throughout this book.

There also have been a few medical doctors that I have worked with on different matters, all great folks. One was a blacksmith friend of mine. The reason I mention this fellow is that he treated a lot of people right from his livery stable, using modern medicines that were available at the time, mixed in with natural herbs.

He told me one time that we are people who thrive on explanations.

Today I have one excellent Doctor friend, which I came to know after moving here to Port Loring. Dr. Graham Wood. He is not just your everyday doctor, far from it. He is kind, takes time for his patients and has a great personality. He has always been there for my family and me when needed, and I have never seen him get angry. Although, I suspect he does raise an eyebrow now and then when someone isn't taking the right road to a healthy lifestyle.

I have asked him to write a bit about his views on Natural Medicines, which I will add later.

Remember, life is made up of choices, whether it be happiness or suffering. Myself I like to think on the happy side of things and nothing can be more joyful than Nature.

When starting out using Nature do not rush into things, or try to do things all at once. Start off by looking at oneself, then making lifestyle changes, like eating habits being changed, lots of exercises and fresh air, with lots of good water.

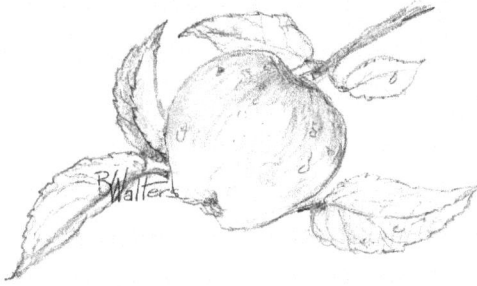

Getting Started

The first thing on the list is to become aware of what is good and bad in your diet. This book tells you that. So now what to do with all that information! I know it is overwhelming at first, but broken down to daily living it becomes natural.

The first thing is to make a list of the regular meals you eat weekly. Are they packaged food or do you make them yourself? Most packaged food is quite easy and quick to make yourself from scratch.

Pick out your most favourite meals and see how you can make them healthier. Changing just a few things in your recipes can make a huge difference in your health. Like changing the oil you use, the way you heat it, the pots or dishes you make it in.

Here are a few suggestions which can start you on your way to a healthier you and family too! Replace regular sugar with organic coconut palm sugar. Use organic extra virgin (cold pressed) olive oil in dressing. Use organic butter or organic coconut oil to replace all other oils. Replace half your food on your supper plate with a tossed salad or steamed vegetables.

When wanting a sweet fix...choose fresh fruit or 70% cocoa pure dark chocolate. The vegetables and fruit that have the most nutrition are bright-coloured. Choose more of these. Find a few new healthy recipes to try to add to your week. Variety is the key to happy eating.

Prepare a grocery list ahead of time so you have everything on hand that you will need. Night time snacks? Nuts and fruit are an excellent choice for that or air-popped popcorn with coconut oil. Tastes Great!

Adding a few different spices to your dishes will give it a whole new flavour and health benefits. Variety again. Having a glass of room temperature water with freshly squeezed lemon juice every morning helps your liver get rid of all the toxins in your body, which in turn helps your immune system.

You can also add nutrition to your breakfast cereal by adding a few raw sunflower seeds, ground flax seeds and some fruit. I add raspberries, bananas and blueberries to mine. A few sunflower seeds and Thompson seedless raisins added to a salad is also a tasty idea.

Trying a few of these suggestions will make a world of difference in your body. You will feel more energized, happier, wanting to do more. A nice healthy walk first thing in the morning is also an excellent beginning for the day. It helps clear the mind and fill your lungs with lots of fresh air.

If you can't find the time for that, park your car the farthest away from the door at work, go outside to eat your lunch if you can. If going shopping, again park in the parking lot the farthest away. Getting sunshine and fresh air is that easy. No Gym equipment needed.

Replace your shampoo and cream rinse and cleaning products with good old baking soda and vinegar. Save a lot of $. Vinegar and baking soda also softens and freshens clothing in your wash.

By giving your body the nutrition, exercise, fresh air and sunshine it needs, your body can fix itself. Be patient! It took a lot of years to get that way. In the end, you will get to know your body, what helps it and what doesn't.

Make changes slowly. Your body needs time to adjust. With all these good things being given, they will be busy fixing and healing, making new happier healthier cells to get you on the road to recovery.

One more suggestion I would like to add. A daily diary of what you have changed and how you feel would be a great asset. That way when someone asks you. "What have you been doing? You look wonderful!" You will be able to tell them.

I do hope you will try these suggestions as I am sure you will feel better, have more energy and the whole family will benefit. These are all things we can do for ourselves and less time spent in the doctor's office.

" Life is Good!"

By: Ruth Walters

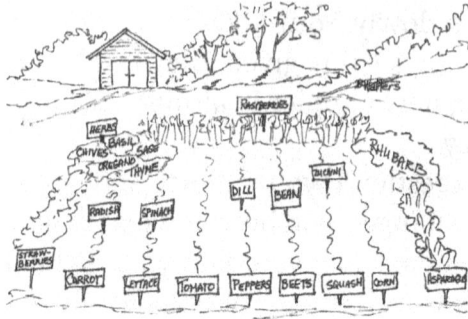

Nutrition

Nutrition is where health begins.

The body is a vessel that transports us around, something like your car. If you don't do your oil changes, it stops running. Same goes for your body, as it also needs constant maintenance.

Our body is quite amazing. In spite of what we put in it or on it, it sorts things out the best way it can and seeks to survive. Most though take their body for granted, by subjecting it to unhealthy things.

Take our chemicals today. If a person looked around, they would see they surround us. Compounds are found in clothes, water, food, air, and lots more. Let's take a look at one biggie in my eyes.

Plastic; Plastic has entered our lives without anyone taking notice. Today it is found everywhere. Most plastics arrive through the petroleum industry. Some though are made using plant-based substances, one being glucose. Unfortunately, converting the stuff into usable forms remains a complicated process. Still, it is an option, and one that I hope is pursued.

For now though plastic is everywhere which I believe is one of the leading causes of our poor health today. So what is one to do? I think we should be looking towards purchasing glass if at all possible.

My wife and I have been striving every day to eliminate plastics from our home in the way of food storage and cooking. We have found that using mason jars is an economical solution for storing items, and they also work quite well to freeze things in if care is taken.

To eliminate all plastics throughout the house might seem next to impossible. But you can take steps to eliminate the ones that are the most dangerous to our health. I believe they are in our food department.

Until you come up with your agenda in removing plastics from your home here are a few suggestions. One thing that will help immensely health-wise is not to cook using plastic-wrap or store hot foods in any plastic whatsoever. When some plastics are subjected to heat, I believe it then releases the toxic chemical called Bisphenol-A (BPA), a potent hormone disruptor.

Truth be known we have been subjected to these substances for several years, without anything being done about it, other than putting a label on specific items stating it is there. Better than nothing I suppose, but still not enough.

It seems to me there is a lot of that going on today. Like pesticides in and on our food or antibiotics. They say they are safe to eat as long as they are low in quantities. Again think about this. Are they safe to eat?

I don't know about you, but those few words should put up red flags. My friends, I don't believe for one minute that any pesticides are safe to eat. None whatsoever.

Now comes the antibiotics. In some instances, I believe they are beneficial, work quite well, and have saved a lot of lives. Antibiotics, as I said, have helped millions of people, but I believe they have also contributed to making millions of people and animals sick, mostly from mismanagement.

My theory on the subject of why so many folks take them is this. I believe that most of our minds have been corrupted into thinking that whatever certain organizations and powers-that-be say is taken as the truth; without giving it a second thought or doing any research to find out different.

It doesn't take a scientist to see these things. It is right in front of us. My favourite way of explaining to folks about this is as follows:

Years ago we had two Clydesdales, yes horses. These two horses would work their hearts out for us at any given time, day or night. But a problem was born. With so much going on around us while working, they got distracted.

Here is where it got interesting. We added blinders on each side of the horses' eyes. This stopped them from seeing what was happening from the broad perspective, keeping them only seeing what was in front of them. Meaning, what we wanted them to see. With the blinders, these horses now did exactly what we wanted them to do.

So do you get my point? Well if not here it is. We have been put into horse-mode. Blinders have been put on our eyes, so we can't see what is happening around us. We have been fooled into seeing and believing only what these powers-that-be want us to see.

So, my friends, that is the one reason why I am writing this book. It is time now to take the blinders off. Take control of your own life and look around. It's an amazing world we live in, with so much to offer other than what the powers-that-be want for us. In doing so, I believe you will begin living a life that is beyond one's imagination.

Now that is out-of-the-way, let us get back to the nutritional side of things. With plastics slowly being eliminated you now should be directing your thoughts on what you should be eating.

First, you have to find out where the body is; pH now comes into the picture. Test yourself, see where you're at, then we can go shopping.

For years, I hated to go shopping as it seemed to me that all I was accomplishing was the elimination of money from my wallet. Then later I found that what I was buying wasn't that good health-wise, for my family or me. Today when I go to buy something I look at the package where it says ingredients. If the product does not provide ingredient information or has words I cannot pronounce, my instincts say, don't buy it.

Now let's take a look at fibre. There are all kinds of health issues, from saying you need good fibre in your diet for good health, where others say that you don't need any fibre at all, as it is a natural substance which arrives from all kinds of plants. The main ingredient in many fibres is called Inulin. It doesn't sound too impressive, but it is an excellent item to get my message across.

I believe today that companies have used the word and item to increase their sales, and they do it quite well. How do they do this? Well, simple really, it all boils down to information put in such a way that we think it is a good thing when it isn't.

So let's get a bit more into Inulin. Inulin is a natural storage carbohydrate present in more than 36,000 species of plants. Inulin is increasingly used in processed foods because it has unusually adaptable characteristics. Its flavour ranges from bland to subtly sweet (approx. 10% sweetness of sugar/sucrose). It can be used to replace sugar, fat, and flour. This is advantageous because Inulin contains 25-35% of the food energy of carbohydrates (starch, sugar).

In addition to being a versatile ingredient, Inulin has many health benefits. Inulin increases calcium absorption and possibly magnesium absorption while promoting the growth of beneficial intestinal bacteria. Chicory Inulin is reported to increase absorption of calcium in girls and lower calcium absorption in men. So why have I gotten so in depth with Inulin? Truth is Inulin is very important to one maintaining a healthy body.

What happens is these companies take a much-needed substance derived from Nature and now reproduce it on its own and put it together with products that aren't natural. In doing so, folks see the word Inulin on the label thinking they got a product that is loaded with a substance that is good for them when in essence it isn't.

Naturally found in plants, a person can eat pretty well as much as they want. But now they have isolated the Inulin or extracted it, and are adding it to all kinds of products like candy, chocolate bars, drinks, fibre-less yogourt and all sorts of snacks. Now, you start eating more than your body can tolerate and problems start, like gastrointestinal issues.

The point is that it isn't just Inulin that they are doing this with; it is thousands of other items.

Today when my wife and I go shopping it is a happy event. We still spend money, probably more so than when we were not eating so well. But without proper health, what have we got? The main aisles we head for is the produce section. These aisles could pretty well sustain most of our bodies' needs to function in a healthy state.

Here your body is smiling while walking along. It knows that health is coming its way. The smells alone in this section tell the body that it's going to be a great day.

Most times though the body is let down, as it is forced to enter the other aisles, where it knows hesitantly that it is going to be subjected to items that contain chemicals, by-products, GMOs, or other harmful ingredients. Right away it starts to feel sick.

This sick feeling is where a person should start to realize that something is wrong. This is the gift that I will share with you throughout the book.

The mind over the years now realizes that it should start taking notice that if it doesn't look after the body, it is in for some hard times. In the beginning, while the body gets established, the brain puts it through all kinds of unhealthy things. Then things change. The body starts sending serious messages to the brain saying, HEY! What are you doing to me? If this keeps up, we are both going to cease-to-exist. You can't keep putting these things into me or on me and expect me to feel good.

So how do I go about correcting this inadequate way of life?

First off, take out your grocery list and scratch off any processed foods. Then comes generic multi-vitamins, soy, soy protein, tofu and soy milk, artificial sweeteners, whole grain cereal, canola oil, low-sodium or healthy choice soups, light and sugar-free salad dressings.

I also have noticed that a lot of folks are into buying canned goods thinking this is an excellent way of getting some good healthy items into the body. I believe this is another reason why our bodies are feeling so poorly. We can't blame the food that is inside the cans, but what isn't nourishing is what they are adding to the food, like preservatives and things. If not bad enough, they now line the cans with plastic.

I can see their reasoning for adding these linings, as with the cans being made from aluminum and other products, they figured they should come up with something to protect us. I believe they replaced it with a sleeping giant that is now coming alive in everyone's body. I feel that this giant is going to be a little harder to slay than Jack had to do in Jack & The Beanstalk. A story that I have enjoyed many times over growing up.

Going back to good old glass jars I would think would help our food industry immensely.

Next is a list of what I believe should be in that grocery cart once it reaches the checkout. I realize that it would be a bit expensive to buy all these in one trip to the market, but we have to start somewhere.

Almonds, apples, asparagus, avocado, banana, beets, black-strap molasses, blueberries, brazil nuts, broccoli, cabbage, cantaloupe, carrots, cashews, cauliflower, celery, cherries, dark chocolate, citrus fruit, coconut, cranberries, cucumbers, dates, eggs, figs, flaxseed, grape seeds, grapes, green beans, green bell peppers, organic honey, honeydew melon, kale, kiwi, leeks, lemons, lentils, lettuce, lima beans, lime, mango, maple syrup, mushrooms, mustard, oat bran, oats, olive oil, onions, oranges, peaches, pears, peas, pecans, pine nuts, pineapples, potatoes, radishes, raspberries, red cabbage, red wine for cooking, rye, sea salt, sea vegetables, sesame seeds, shiitake mushrooms, snow peas, spinach, strawberries, sunflower seeds, sweet potatoes, tomatoes, walnuts, watermelon, wheat germ and zucchini.

Keep in mind when looking at this list that whenever possible make sure you buy organic. You could look at starting your own garden, which I believe more folks should be doing.

I do have a gardening book out there called "Join Me In The Garden" that deals with how to get that vegetable garden started and maintaining it. Along with all kinds of tips, recipes and things that my Father, Grandfather, Laura, Reg, Grey Wolf and myself learned over the years. Great book.

Now don't get to thinking that I am out just to sell books, as I am not. My main objective here is to get the word out of how important it is for one to become and stay healthy. If we don't look after the body, we without a doubt will have to undergo some real hardships. Which is unnecessary.

There have been scores of people that have asked me, "how do you know what works and what doesn't." I have watched, listened, done significant research throughout my life, talked to doctors of all kinds, natural and modern-day, along with experimenting on my own. But most of all, I was lucky enough to have some great folks throughout my life share with me what they had learned.

Over the years I watched them heal folks using only the plants and things that grew around them. With a lot of common sense thrown in for good measure. They were terrific people, just wanting to help those in need, asking nothing in return.

On common sense, my wife and I were talking to our son Karl one time, and he said that for most things in life, common sense is what a lot of people use the least of nowadays, whereas it should be on top of the list in priorities. I agree wholeheartedly with those few words. Smart young man as both my sons are; we are very proud of them.

Then there are those that have said I have grown strong in body and spirit, along with being active in my strive to live the old ways. I have to say they are right.

Some have said that I shouldn't be suggesting that there are other options for treating diseases. As in doing so, I could cause great grief if the treatments using Nature didn't work. They have even taken it further and said how can I know what it's like to have cancer or other illnesses. So how do I answer these folks?

In all sincerity, I don't like to talk about issues relating to myself. But since a lot have asked, here is my answer.

I did have biopsies taken from inside my body in 2010, and yes, they did find cancer. Was I upset? Well, sure I was, as anyone would be. So scared I had to pull the car off to the side of the road coming home from the doctor's office, as I got to shaking so bad I couldn't hold onto the wheel. The only thing that brought me back to normal or what one could call normal at that time was my lovely wife. She was there to hold my hand and listen to the words that at that moment along that old highway, probably should not have been said or heard by no one. It was a release, as it were, and what was needed.

She listened without saying a word, comforting me as needed and we then proceeded home. Not one more word was said the rest of that day from her or myself. We both needed time to digest the new information that was bestowed upon us both.

Then later that night my body went into profound cold sweats. My heart and body felt like nothing I have ever felt all the days of my life. For most of the night my body went through convulsions, shaking so violently that I thought I was going to die. Here once again my wife came to my side and with no words, just her presence, I settled down.

For a week I thrashed things around in my mind of what I should do. It wasn't easy.

Then, my very good friend and doctor, Graham Wood dropped by to see how I was doing. We sat at the table, and he took the time to explain in great detail exactly what, if I decided to, the modern day treatments would consist of and how they would go about the procedures through surgery and then radiation along with other things afterwards.

I have to say it didn't help my nerves any whatsoever at the time. We talked some more, and I then told him straight man to man that there is no way that I was going to subject my body to these treatments or more so, my family.

He smiled, and with that, he said he would be there for me no matter what.

You know, those few words were the tipping of the scale in which way I chose to go. Just knowing he would be there if I needed him was the inspiration that made things happen that day.

From there the days passed, and I didn't want to talk about it anymore. I didn't want to even take into account that I had cancer. I just wanted it to go away.

Of course, it wouldn't or couldn't, as I had things to do. I had first to get a grip on my life. In other words, take control of my life back. I then got to talking to folks that had cancer, spoke to hundreds of them. Listened to how they were treating it, what the side effects were, how much they had suffered emotionally and internally. Most not very nice. But it had to be done. I had to expose myself and see what this disease, as they now call it, was all about, how it played out in the body, what it was made of and what caused it to begin with. What caused it was the way to getting better which I found out a year or so later.

I then proceeded to the Internet and read, read, read and read some more. I read both sides of the story a thousand times over. Meaning treating it with modern-day ways along with natural means. To make a long story short, I chose natural —or should say Nature.

Now here is what separates me from most others. I now put in motion a plan. First off, no more reading about the treatments of today. I do of course keep an eye on anything new coming down the road, but so far there is nothing other than the same old treatments that they have been using for fifty years.

Not pleasant, nor do I think it is right what they are subjecting folks' bodies to. There is no way that anyone—and I mean this, anyone—can make me believe that by poisoning the body with all kinds of deadly chemicals or slicing it up like a cucumber, or by burning one's insides until nothing can function on its own, is the correct way of dealing with this.

So now with this in mind, I put everything into perspective. Weighing everything and I mean everything and everyone's opinion, it was quite clear on what I had to do. Using Nature, becoming part of her, was the answer.

For years now I have seen some pretty amazing things take place in my body. All good. Just one more reason or reasons for writing this book as I hope it helps others that have been given this kind of news. I want them to realize that there are alternatives and other options and that literally hundreds if not thousands of others are and have been treating cancer and other diseases successfully, using nothing less than what in most cases is right outside your front door.

If there is any part that you don't understand why I chose this road, well, you haven't been listening. My friends, the choice is yours and yours alone. Which is the way it should be.

Getting Better: The single and most important way of treating any ailment is first we have to find the cause. Without doing that how can we fix things? It is impossible.

It came to me that the lifestyle I was living made me sick, simple as that. So with that set in my mind I now knew that if I wanted to get better, I would have to make some drastic changes.

Nutrition top of the list, then on to eliminating stress from all avenues, exercise, lots of sunshine for vitamin D and other good things and lots of good fresh water to flush out the bad. Along with adding natural treatments that I know to be wholesome and true.

In doing so, I got better. Today I feel great, healthy, wanting to do things in life and looking forward to each day. Set your mind right the first thing in the morning and the rest becomes easy.

So now when someone asks, "how do you know your way is right?" I just smile and say, "Look at me, do I look like someone that is down and out. I am standing here before you with a smile on my face looking and feeling fantastic. No more pain, no worry, life is good."

There are, however, some that say no it doesn't. With that I smiled and taken from a phrase a good friend told me one time, I say this. "Why should the way I feel be dependent on what others think?"

The use of Nature wasn't just brought on with me finding out I had cancer. Throughout my life, I was subjected to lots of other things, like bad teeth where the pain was so severe I would scream at night for it to stop. Swellings of the mouth around the teeth so severely full of poison that I had to take all kinds of antibiotics to stay alive. The solution: finally getting the nerve up to have them all taken out and once done using Nature, I managed to get myself back on track.

Hernias for most of my life, one fixed by modern-day treatments which has troubled me all my life, as it wasn't done right. I was also subjected to waking up on the operating table, as their sleeping compound somehow didn't work right, or wasn't administered right. I still wake up some nights in cold sweats looking around for my Dad to help me. In time I found plants and barks from trees that helped with this problem.

Others were broken wrists brought on by someone that pushed me down some stairs. For years, I was in pain only to be relieved by natural ointments given to me by my old Native Friend Grey Wolf.

Eye problems like a cataract that started to cover my right eye to be cleared up by simply picking some raspberry leaves, mixing it with some rose petals and rinsing out my eyes once a day.

Back problems where others were put on disability for life. Using Nature, I found cures that took the pain away and got me moving again doing what I loved.

Hip needed to be replaced, where I sought out the properties in a plant called comfrey and applied it faithfully every day until the pain disappeared.

Arthritis and Rheumatism entered my body caused by overwork throughout my life; the pain was relieved by using different plants made into ointments, tinctures and infusions.

Stomach Ulcer where I had to undergo endoscopy many times. The ulcer wasn't half as bad as what the endoscopy did to me, as my body went into awful spasms and my colon still goes into them today if I get upset.

It was quite painful, but with a little research trying different things, I pretty well eased the problem when the spasms occurred, using nothing but good clean water, sipping a wee bit at a time.

Then in finding the ulcer which consisted of 3/4 of my stomach, they said it would have to be operated on, or I would be in dire trouble. I said give me some time. With that, they said until I came back for the operation to take Tagamet (an ulcer drug) that was just coming on the market back then. I did, but it made me feel sick. For the longest time, I suffered.

Then new drugs came on-line, proton inhibitors. To sum this up, I took thousands of them, with the doctors at the time saying I will be on them the rest of my life.

My wife was at her wit's end as there was no way she could make me anything to eat that didn't bother my stomach. Got so bad I was in the bathroom more than working. Pain so bad sometimes it buckled me over.

Then one day after years of suffering I got talking to another Native friend of mine. He told me about taking probiotics. I listened and started to take four a day in the beginning, eating lots of veggies for the enzymes, as both are needed for a healthy stomach.

With a lot of withdrawals and some significant pain going off the treatments they prescribed, I finally started feeling better. Bloating, gas, major pain slowly all went away. Every day got better and better. I began to enjoy life again, thanks to Nature.

Just before writing this book I started once again to have some stomach problems. With the knowledge I had gained from an earlier time, I was able to narrow it down that an ulcer was starting to form once again in my stomach. I didn't need any x-ray or endoscopy to tell me what was wrong. I knew from experiences of long ago.

I talked to my very good friend Dr. Wood about it, and he said I could have my blood tested for H. pylori, which I thought was a good idea at the time, as H. pylori is a great contributor to stomach ulcers.

Then I got to looking at some of Grey Wolf's notes and found that he treated hundreds of folks for stomach ulcers using nothing more than cabbage juice. The results were astounding, he said.

So my wife and I decided on buying a really good juicer, which we did. We then got to juicing up some cabbage—red, purple and green. Almost immediately I had good reports coming in from my stomach. Within two days the pain started to leave. Within two weeks I was pretty well back to normal.

What happens is the cabbage juice kills H. pylori; along with that it is very alkaline, which is what is needed for healing the stomach. Acid I believe is what causes the pain by burning the sore areas of the stomach. Cabbage juice reduces the acid levels plus coats the walls of the stomach, thus allowing the stomach to heal. Nothing could be simpler.

I took about 3 ounces or so a 1/2 hour after I ate breakfast, another 3 ounces 1/2 hour after lunch and another 3 ounces just before going to bed.

I could keep on writing about different ailments all looked at by the medical profession. Truth be known, hardly any of them was cured using the treatments or drugs they put me on—not one. I will say this though; they did help with the pain which allowed me to continue with my life for a spell.

So what does all this mean? My views are that over the years with all these things happening I should have seen what was being shown to me.

An explanation would go something like this. A fellow goes into a bar. On his way out there is another fellow that hits him over the head with a baseball bat. If one is smart, he doesn't go back out that door ever again. But for me I kept going back out that door, knowing fully well the fellow was out there waiting. I kept on doing it without a second thought.

What was shown to me was that I had to find another road.

If I had taken the time to research this earlier in life and seen what Nature was trying to show me, I could have fixed the problem once and for all and saved myself a lot of grief and pain. I didn't; I was like most others, I had blinders on.

Today I see things more clearly and know that for 75% of all our sickness and ordeals through life, most can be fixed by turning to Nature and changing one's lifestyle. Also, the most things I worried about never took place.

I believe today they treat symptoms only. They don't take the time to find out the cause, or for that matter sit and listen to the patient. Not all though, as there are a few that recognize and act accordingly. I have some very good friends in the medical profession and take what they have to say to heart. They're very hard to find, but they are out there.

My research shows most can't see that the reason for cancer is that a malfunction in our system causes it. It needs to be corrected and cries for us to do so.

Finally, here are two lists of foods. The reason I am mentioning them is that some foods have more chemicals on them than others. These below are my choice that I feel should be taken into consideration when buying.

These Should Always Be Organic:
Apples, celery, cherry tomatoes, cucumbers, grapes, hot peppers, nectarines if imported, peaches, potatoes, spinach, strawberries, sweet bell peppers, kale/collard greens and summer squash.

Choices If Not Organic:
Asparagus, avocados, cabbage, cantaloupe, sweet corn, *(not to be confused with potentially GMO canned corn)* eggplant, grapefruit, kiwi, mangoes, mushrooms, onions, papayas, pineapples, sweet peas and sweet potatoes.

I would also like to mention that if you can not get fresh vegetables, frozen would be a better choice rather than vegetables in a can.

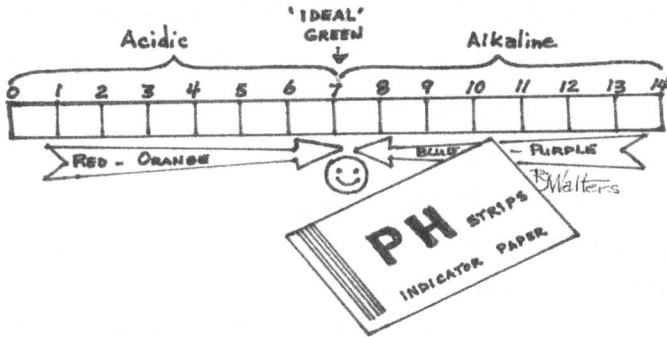

Acidic 'IDEAL' GREEN Alkaline

0 1 2 3 4 5 6 7 8 9 10 11 12 13 14

RED – ORANGE BLUE – PURPLE

BWalters

PH STRIPS INDICATOR PAPER

pH

Let's start by saying this. "It is pretty hard to treat something if one doesn't know where they are health-wise." I would think everyone would agree with that, right? Then let's get on to talking about one's pH. The pH of one's body other than the blood should sit between 7 - 7.6 which is a touch alkaline.

The pH scale goes from 0 to 14 with 7 being neutral. Everything below that is acid, everything above is alkaline. While talking about pH, I would like to say this for those of us that had or is dealing with cancer.

Naturally, when dealing with cancer conditions, it's best to work with a trusted health-care professional with a proven track record of success in treating cancer naturally. Always ask the hard questions of your medical provider, don't be manoeuvred into doing things you don't want, it's your life on the line!

I genuinely believe that we are looking in the wrong direction if we think we can outmanoeuvre the body. I believe that cancer is not a disease at all, it instead is a healing process. In other words, a wake-up call that something needs to be done and done quickly. In most cases, after initiating a healthy lifestyle, it either disappears or moves into a dormant, harmless state. The fact of the matter is, if you have a healthy body you don't have cancer or any other disease.

So what does all this mean, in the way we stay healthy or get healthy? "This is where pH comes into play." We now have to check our pH and see where we are at. Once we know this, we can move forward. The way to do this is to use a pH test kit or strips you can buy online or from your health food provider. It is just a strip of litmus paper that turns colour. They come in a box with instructions and pictures of where you are at when you check your pH.

The best time to check your pH is in the morning before you have eaten or drank anything. I check my urine first then my saliva. Always swallow a mouth full of saliva first then do the test, as overnight acids have a way of building up and a correct reading will not be able to be established. Your urine will usually be a touch more acidic than your saliva.

I should also mention here that your blood pH always stays the same sitting at 7.35 - 7.45. The pH of the human digestive tract, however, varies greatly and is entirely different, this is the pH you want to keep in check. Reason being the body will do whatever it has to, to maintain the blood pH where it is supposed to be. If it didn't, we would die.

If our body were healthy, it wouldn't have to rob things from places that it shouldn't. Now you know where you are. If too alkaline you eat more acidic foods. If too acidic you eat more alkaline foods. Easy & quick. With the rinsing of your veggies in Organic Apple Cider Vinegar you not only do all that I stated above, but you also raise your pH, as it is very alkalizing; but this just isn't enough.

Research shows that most diseases today including cancer is brought on by the body being too acidic. The remedy is to check pH and go from there. If one thinks about it, our bodies are the same as the soil we walk on. Why? Well if one wants to grow edible crops, the soil needs to be kept in the 7.5 range, the same as our body.

pH Food Guide

Next are two lists. The first being from the Highest Alkaline to the Lowest Alkaline forming foods. Then from the Highest Acids to the Lowest Acid forming foods. Great list to have on hand when trying to get your pH into the right perspective.
Alkaline Forming Foods

—Highest Alkaline
—Baking Soda, Sea Salt, Mineral Water.
—Spinach, Chard, Kale, Dandelion Greens.
—Lemons, Watermelon, Limes, Grapefruit.
—High Alkaline
—Carrots, Celery, Lettuce, Zucchini.
—Dates, Figs, Raisins, Melons.
—Almonds, Chestnuts, Herbal Teas.

—Low Alkaline
—Apples, Pears, Peaches, Bananas.
—Green Beans, Cauliflower, Cabbage.
—Apple Cider Vinegar, Quinoa, Wild Rice.
—Lowest Alkaline
—Avocado, Coconut Oil, Flax Oil.
—Cherries, Tomatoes, Potatoes (with skin).
—Millet, Lentils, Fresh Corn.
Acid Forming Foods

—Highest Acid
—Antibiotics, Processed Sugar, Cocoa.
—Beef, Pork, Shellfish, Fried Foods.
—Processed Cheese, Jams, Jellies, Liquor.
—High Acid
—Chicken, Veal, Organ Meats.
—Beer, Wine, Sweetened Fruit Juice.

—White Flour, Pastries, Peanuts.

—Low Acid
—Turkey, Lamb, Wild Duck, Venison.
—Soft Drinks, Coffee, Black Tea.
—White Rice, Soy Milk, Aged Cheese.
—Lowest Acid
—Brown Rice, Oats, Rye.
—Fish, Eggs, Yogurt.
—Honey, Maple Syrup, Canola Oil.

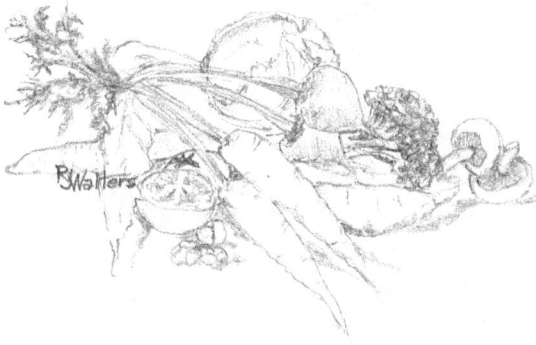

Probiotics

One remedy sold years ago was a pill made up by naturalists called the Vegetable-Pill. Fixed pretty well any stomach problems one might have. What was in that magic pill? Well, it's like what we have today really, just named differently. Today we call the tablets probiotics.

They are in reality millions of tiny live bacteria, which we need in our stomach and intestines to survive. With all the antibiotics being taken today in our foods and medicines we have killed most of them, which in return has caused a lot of health-related issues.

One has to remember that taking probiotics is a good thing, but one also has to remember that there are all kinds of different strains. I think it would be beneficial to chat to your doctor or a well reputable naturalist and come up with a plan that would be best for you. I cannot stress enough how important these bacteria are.

Years ago I had a major ulcer. I had endoscopies and was put on all kinds of medication. In the beginning, they helped some, but after taking them for a while, all my symptoms returned.

So one day while looking at some notes that Grey Wolf put together I noticed one where he talked about my problem. I decided that I would change a few things. I started taking probiotics daily. Things then began to improve. With that happening, after chatting with my doctor friend, I slowly took myself off of the medicines that I was taking.

The only thing I do now and then if things don't seem just right in my stomach, is change the type of bacteria to a new strain. Easy to do and problem solved.

Good live bacteria can be found in pill form, and some yogurt, but it's my opinion that yogurt isn't as good as taking it by itself. You can also get it from eating lots of green raw vegetables or making your own sauerkraut.

After Probiotics, one should take a close look at what they are eating. I would say today that folks should be eating 70% vegetables and 30% good meat, meaning free range or pesticide and hormone free. More and more organics are coming to your local supermarket as each day passes. If not where you shop, ask for it.

While on the topic of vegetables and fruits. Today they are coming in from all different countries, especially throughout the winter months. My wife and I do a lot of canning and freezing using our own from our gardens which I recommend to anyone that has the means to do so. Nothing is healthier for you than homegrown or locally grown produce.

So what can you do to make not so good produce into healthy produce? With all the chemicals that are on our produce, it is a challenge.

I also found there is a parasite on some vegetables that can cause a lot of grief, flu-like symptoms. Apple cider vinegar to the rescue as it can kill this parasite and helps remove chemicals.

My wife takes the fresh raw vegetables from our garden or supermarket and lets them soak in a large bowl of water mixed with some organic apple cider vinegar while she gets the rest of the meal ready. It amounts to two tablespoons to one gal of water. A little is fine. Once she has everything else prepared, she then rinses the vegetables in cold water and makes the salad. We found this to be very helpful.

Another thing I have found is that anxiety, meaning stress from work, home, family, friends, money, all and more can cause a lot of digestive problems. The good news is that by taking a few probiotics throughout the day can help your digestive system get back to normal.

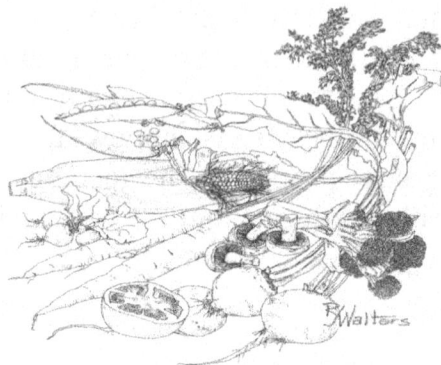

Cholesterol

Cholesterol seems today, has been made into such a bad thing. Causes hundreds of different problems. But does it? I honestly believe there is no such thing as Bad Cholesterol or Good Cholesterol. The only thing there is is Cholesterol.

I was going to write a bit on the subject but a friend of mine, Allan Lawry wrote one of the best articles relating to Cholesterol that I have ever read. So I asked him if he would mind me putting his article in the book for all to read. He happily agreed.

It explains everything in an easy-to-understand way. Take a look.

"Bad" cholesterol: the unknown heart healer
by Allan Lawry

Source: HANS e-News - February 15, 2012

If you think that "bad" or "high" cholesterol contributes to heart disease, you have been deceived by those marketing a mythical disease.

The so-called "bad" or LDL cholesterol is actually part of a natural healing process designed for repairing damaged arteries in your body. This damage is usually caused by inflammation and oxidation. Oxidation causes nicks and cuts on the inside of the walls of the arteries and causes inflammation, similar to a cut on the outside of your skin. This then sets into motion the process of healing. LDL cholesterol has many purposes, and one of them is to assist in the healing process by forming a waxy "scab" over the cuts that still allows blood to flow smoothly. Often called plaque this scab gives the arterial wall's protection and time to heal from within.

It is up to us as the owners of those arteries to provide the correct ingredients for the initial healing process and to create healthy arteries for a lifetime.

The myths of cholesterol need to be understood. Many studies show that people with high cholesterol live longer and have fewer heart conditions than those with low cholesterol and that high cholesterol does not predict all-cause mortality either. Studies also show that if you eat fatty foods that contain high levels of cholesterol it has little or no effect on changes in blood cholesterol levels.

So, in reality, there is no reason to describe it as being high or low, good or bad, as explained by Ron Rosedale, MD. "Notice please that LDL and HDL are lipoproteins which are fats combined with proteins. There is only one cholesterol. There is no such thing as "good" or "bad" cholesterol; there is just cholesterol."

Years ago, mainstream medicine noticed that the "bad" LDL cholesterol showed up in higher amounts with people who had various heart conditions. Thinking this was one of the causes of the problems, they hypothesized that high LDL levels in the blood were a major risk factor for heart conditions. They did not do their homework and did not realize that LDL shows up to "patch" the holes and cracks inside the arterial walls.

It has since been found that those who proposed the lowering of LDL levels were being paid by the drug companies who were producing the cholesterol-lowering drugs. In my 30 years as a healthy living coach I have seen the level lowered three times by these so-called "experts!"

Dr.Uffe Ravnskov (MD, Ph.D.) is a leading cholesterol researcher who was recently asked.

"If the cholesterol hypothesis is an error, does this mean that all therapies, low cholesterol diets, cholesterol-lowering therapies, and medications are wrong?" His response; "Absolutely, this kind of treatment is meaningless, costly and has transformed millions of healthy people into patients."

The most common drugs currently given out for "high cholesterol" are called statins, and they represent a 29 billion dollar business worldwide. They work by inhibiting an enzyme in the liver that manufactures cholesterol. The medical claim that lowering LDL is beneficial in fighting cardiovascular disease (CVD) is totally contradictory to all the research and results that we have seen for the past 10 years. It is not in your best interest to lower your cholesterol levels!

It is important to understand that cholesterol is an essential and valuable substance for living a healthy life. It is vital for transporting the fat-soluble vitamins A D E, and K. Cholesterol is necessary for forming brain synapses, and it helps to create all sex hormones valuable for a healthy sex life.

To prevent potential CVD, it is essential to lower your exposure to oxidation and inflammation. I suggest a natural, preferably raw and alkaline diet and the avoidance of all refined carbohydrates, refined plant oils and artificial sweeteners. Get plenty of fresh air, exercise and vitamin D from sunshine. Check in with your primary care provider if you are concerned with your levels of intravascular stress (IVS). Procedures include biomarker tests for; elevated C-reactive protein, homocysteine, insulin, glucose and acidosis.

Research has shown that rather than avoiding the so-called "bad fatty cholesterol" the type of fat that needs to be avoided are foods fried in vegetable oils, all hydrogenated oils, refined or processed oils, margarine, trans fats, and any oil that has been overheated. These fats turn rancid and oxidize in the body. This can cause excess free radical production which can cause internal inflammation. Inflammation causes a cascade of problems including the oxidation of LDL cholesterol, a precursor to arterial damage and heart problems such as angina and coronary blockages (heart attacks).

So, the next time you see or hear an advertisement for, lowering your cholesterol, please be aware of the marketing game that is in effect and realize you do not need to buy into their game; your health is more important. I wish you all the best in your quest for a healthier life.

Allan Lawry

I myself years ago was told that things would only get better by taking these drugs.

Didn't take me long to find out that they might have lowered my cholesterol, but they also made every bone in my body ache. I couldn't even lift my arms above my head.

I believed what they told me. Which was, "Precautionary measures, George, it's in your best interest." But was it?

After a few months of pain, I decided to research these drugs. What I found was that all the symptoms I was having were listed as a side effect of the drug I was on. Once known I talked to my doctor, and he said it is up to me if I wanted to stop taking them. I decided then to take myself off the drug. From that day forward things got better, but it did take some time.

You know, I think this is worth mentioning. When I was prescribed them drugs my most inner feelings told me it was wrong. My body and mind were telling me, it wasn't the right thing to do.

Was I so wrong in taking the word of others instead of what my most inner feelings were trying to tell me? Absolutely! As I was taught better, by some pretty impressive people. From that day forward, I followed the instructions that were given to me daily, through my own-self without question.

So what was I to do to improve my health with the subject of cholesterol on my mind?

I learned that cholesterol is the raw material which, through the action of sunshine on the skin, is converted to vitamin D.

So what I decided to do was soak up some sunshine, get lots of exercise, fuel my body with good food and let Nature take its course. Worked for me.

Remember, our bodies respond to every word we speak and to every thought we think.

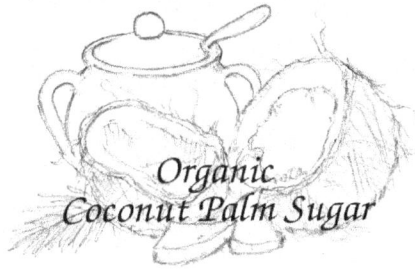

Sugar

White refined sugar is about one of the worst things a person can put into their body. I also don't recommend eating artificial sugars of any kind.

Sugar is in everything today from chewing gum to a glass of milk. Soda pop sits at the top of the list for the highest amounts, and it would be in a person's best interest to drink it with caution. It is stated that it takes a good ten cups of water to flush out just one can of soda from your system.

So what can you use for that sweet tooth? There are other options. Pure maple syrup is one I enjoy now and then. It still has a high sucrose level, which in other words is sugar, but it is a better choice than white sugar and its benefits come directly from Nature herself.

Raw organic honey is another good choice, though the pH is slightly acidic so use it sparingly. Stevia is a natural sweetener you can actually grow yourself. I have done so with great success. The kind my wife and I use is raw organic coconut palm sugar.

Here is something worth knowing. The glycemic index of white sugar sits around 60 and brown sugar around 65. Honey comes in at about 58 and maple syrup at approximately 54. Raw organic coconut palm sugar however comes in at 35, which means it does not give the blood a sharp sugar spike like all the rest. It is quite expensive, but what is good health worth?

My theory on the whole is this. Refined white sugar is about the worst of the bunch, and the artificial sweeteners on the market today are not far behind. Research suggests that excess sugar interferes with the ability of white blood cells to fight bacteria and depletes calcium, one of the body's most needed minerals. Just a few more reasons to watch your sugar intake.

And here is something a lot of folks don't realize. Carbs are sugar too. Question: What may be the single healthiest choice you can make? Answer: Choose to never eat calorie-dense carbohydrates. Question: Calorie-dense carbohydrates? What's that? Answer: Any form of rice, any form of corn, any form of potato, and anything made from wheat — bread, donuts, cookies, crackers, chips, pretzels, and everything else. In other words, any grain or starch based food.

Question: Whoa there. That seems rather extreme. Besides, I like cookies. And what about whole grain? I thought that was good for me. Answer: This is a complex topic and it is controversial, not because there is much doubt about it any longer, but because it is not what anyone, including me, wants to discover is true. But I am afraid that it is. Question: What if I just back off on those things a bit? Answer: That does not work at all. Perhaps you have tried that in the past. It needs to be total avoidance or don't bother. Amazing things happen if you can get over onto the other side of the Sugar Hill. And it is a bit of a hill to climb.

You have the ability of choosing, I hope you choose wisely.

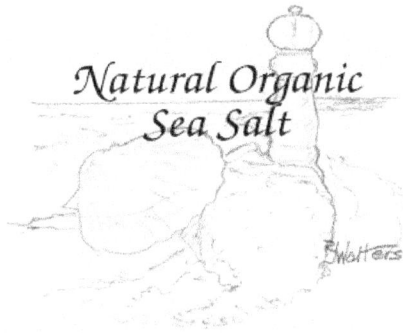

Salt

Salt I feel has been given a bad rap. Why is that? Well, salt is one of the leading ingredients of keeping a body healthy. Without salt, we would become quite ill.

It's not the salt that is bad for you; it's the chemicals that they used to refine it with. My wife and I buy natural organic sea salt. When you get this salt, it is greyish, along with being a touch large which my wife grinds. You will have to lay it out at first to dry, as it is a bit damp, which is the way it's supposed to be.

Years ago if you worked in a factory, or where one would work up a sweat, they would have had dispensers that held salt tablets. Reason for this was simple. To maintain proper strong health, and keep up one's strength, salt was needed along with lots of fresh water.

I can't stress enough the importance of getting good healthy salt into one's body. Now in saying this, I should mention that today with all the processed foods which have a very high salt content, one should be a bit careful, and until you wean yourself off all these not so good foods, salt should be used in moderation. Same goes for anything in life.

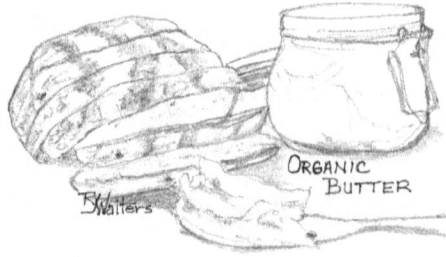
Organic Butter

Butter

Growing up on a dairy farm and producing our cream, butter was always readily available.

Today though butter has been made out to be bad for your health. Is it though? It's my opinion that butter is the best of the best when it comes to one retaining good health.

To start off, it contains high amounts of selenium which is an anti-oxidant.

It also contains iodine which helps stabilize the thyroid gland.

It is rich in vitamin A, which helps with vision and is also a good source of fat-soluble vitamins like E, K and D.

The colon uses butter as an energy source which helps those with constipation and diarrhea.

Finally, note that only natural vitamins like those in butter can be absorbed into the body. Your body can't be fooled, as it knows the difference between natural vitamins and the synthetic ones.

With all this data that is before us, I believe that making a transition back to using; good organic butter would be beneficial to one's health.

In doing so remember this: Salted butter can be left on the counter for four or five days. Unsalted cannot be left on the shelf, as it will go rancid.

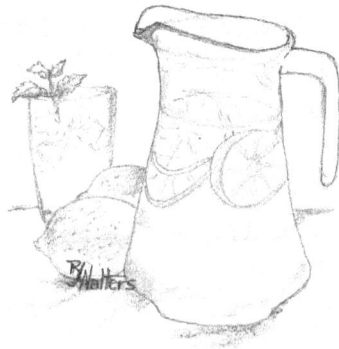

Water

Drinking water is the best thing a person can do in treating all kinds of diseases, along with keeping the body healthy. Drinking water at a certain time I have found maximizes its effectiveness on the body:

2 glasses of water after waking up helps every part of your body get set for the day. 1 glass of water 45 minutes before a meal will help immensely with digestion. 1 glass of water before taking a bath can maintain lower blood pressure. 1 glass of water before going to bed can stop strokes or heart attacks.

I have found that a person should drink eight good glasses of water a day and every day. Reason being our body is made up of mostly water. Without the correct amount, we become sick. I can't say enough about water.

Over the years water has changed drastically, as today most of our tap water is treated in plants with all kinds of chemicals. One is chlorine which I believe does more harm to the body than good. It's a deadly chemical, and my views on the subject are that it should have never been allowed to flow through our water lines. Our officials though say chlorinated tap water is quite safe for humans to drink.

There have been quite a few scientific studies, however, that state that chlorinated tap water is a skin irritant and can be associated with rashes like eczema. This is true too, as here where we live now using only well water I don't have a problem when bathing. But when I go to visit my son in the city and have a shower, two hours later I start to get itchy and in some cases a pretty nasty rash, which takes weeks to eliminate once back home.

As well, the chlorinated water I believe destroys most of our friendly bacteria that help in the digestion of food, which protects the body from harmful diseases. It's worth mentioning that most of these bacteria that the chlorinated water is killing are what we need to stay healthy.

There have also been studies showing that chlorine and chlorinated by-products could be causing instances of bladder, breast and bowel cancer as well as malignant melanoma. Knowing this, I believe that if a person would stop drinking chlorinated water and start drinking natural spring water and taking probiotics, things would soon begin to improve health wise.

Another chemical that is being put in our drinking water today is called fluoride. A study done on this chemical states that fluorides, in general, are toxic to humans, however, Calcium CaF_2 is considered the least toxic, and even relatively harmless due to its extreme insolubility. Moreover, calcium is a well-known antidote for fluoride poisoning. So when a cure exists in combination with a poison, it makes the poison far less toxic to the body. Calcium fluoride is the form of fluoride commonly found in natural, untreated waters.

It is said that sodium Fluorosilicate (Na_2SiF_6) is primarily added to public drinking water as a fluoridation agent. This same compound is also used as an insecticide and a wood preservative. Other names for it are sodium fluosilicate and sodium silica fluoride.

So what is one to do? Millions of folks today drink bottled water, thinking it is the best avenue to getting good water. If I were asked if it was the best route to go, I would have to say no. Reason being I don't much trust the chemicals that are in the plastic bottles.

Some bottled water even has a touch of chlorine and fluoride in it. Also, one doesn't know where the water is coming from. Put that together with a few things that haven't even been found yet, as long-term effects of plastic chemicals, well it's just not right.

I would have to say the best that one could do is to seek out natural springs or someone that has their own well and get your water there. There are a few natural wells in Ontario; one is in Elmvale, Ontario. Right along the highway and easy to get at. Great water, cold and so good for you. Get to Elmvale and ask anyone and they will tell you exactly where it is.

Actually, at the time I wrote this book my wife and I took a drive down to visit some friends and passed the well. What we saw was, they added a nice cement pad and a roof over the top of where the water is running freely. Makes me smile when I see things like this happening.

Here where we live today, we have good water and not a day goes by that eight or so glasses of natural water isn't drunk by my wife and I. It's so cold that you can't hold your hand under the tap, even on the warmest day of summer. We had it tested many times, and it is loaded with all kinds of things which one needs to promote good health throughout the body.

What are other ways out there today for obtaining good water? Well, there are filters and filtration systems, too many to name. A person has to be careful though when purchasing them, as some filters are loaded down with chemicals that aren't good for you. If this is the route you choose to take, ask questions and make sure you get what is right for you. After all, it is your health.

Our farm years ago was spread out over about a hundred acres and along one side of it, there was a valley with a creek running through it. Growing a lot of tender fruit and fresh vegetables, my Dad decided that he would put up a dam at one end of the valley. His thinking was that if we had a really dry year, we would have enough water for irrigation. From that day forward we were never short of good water for all our needs, including a place to fish and swim.

Everyone over the age of 50 has cancer of some sort somewhere in their body, along with many other problems.

Most will never know they exist because their body will cure them all on its own.

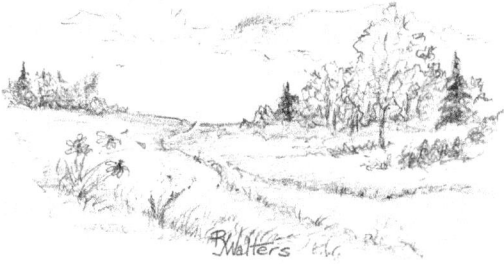

Oxygen

Fresh air, proper breathing. Here is something that we can't live without.

Grey Wolf believed that a lot of the problems folks had health wise could be directly related to the lack of oxygen. What happens is, that if we don't get outside and breathe in good fresh oxygen, our lungs then can't distribute it to our blood cells. If the cells can't get enough oxygen through breathing in fresh air, it turns to an alternate action, called fermentation; which causes the cells to start making a lot of not so good chemicals, which in turn cause unhealthy, weak cells.

If we get the right amount of good oxygen into our system, our cells thrive and can then protect our body from all kinds of diseases, viruses and bacteria that are harmful to us. From all that I have learned I would not hesitate to say that most of all our diseases of today are started by not having enough good clean oxygen.

How does one correct the problem? It's quite simple. Go outside and get some fresh air. If you live in the city, it's my feeling that you should travel outside the city, away from pollutants, such as car exhaust, sewer pipes, the ones that every house has coming up through their roofs, not to forget

43

the ones underground. Let's face it; most folks live in a polluted environment.

One big problem today is that most don't breathe right. Years ago we were taught how to breathe correctly at an early age, but over the years it has been eliminated from our teachings, with the thinking that it is of little concern for one's health. Couldn't be further from the truth.

The proper way to breathe is when you are outside you should bring yourself into a relaxed state. Now expand your stomach slowly, taking in the fresh air at the same time. This allows your lungs to expand inside your chest and you then are capable of bringing in the quantity of air that you are in need of.

On releasing the air, bring your stomach in at the same time. Adding to this, I believe you should breathe in through the nose and out through the mouth. The nose filters the air protecting your lungs from dust and harmful material. Out through the mouth, allows the good properties to stay inside the lungs which promotes good health.

It is a simple process really and comes naturally if practiced. I wouldn't hesitate to say that over three-quarters of the people in the world today, doesn't do it, merely because they weren't taught to do it correctly.

It is also worth mentioning here that oxygen is also a powerful detoxifier, as it is the main ingredient used when it comes to breaking down the excess and toxic materials that are in our bodies. Without good oxygen and the proper amount, your body will become sick.

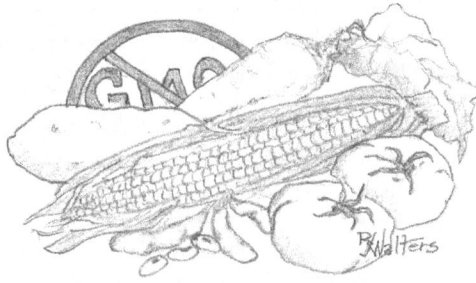

GMO

Genetically Modified Organisms. Everyone should know about GMO. Along with that, everyone should be concerned.

GMO and GE foods are pretty much the same things. They are foods created by merging DNA from different species. Is this a good thing? I believe that we are venturing into a place that no man has gone before.

In reality, GMO foods began in and around 1994. With a chemical called Flavr Savr which was supposed to delay the ripening of tomatoes, giving them longer shelf life in the stores. It didn't pan out though as they thought and other ways and chemicals were created.

Today it's my feeling that things are getting out of hand, as it boils down to just a few major players that have the rights over what seeds are to be planted and what isn't to be planted. Also, the safety of these chemicals and new plants has not been proven, and I believe a lot of our ailments are and will be caused by them in the days to come.

If they are allowed to put these chemicals on or alter the DNA of our food and seeds, then we as the people should have the right to know what foods, plants or seeds they are. It is our right to know, and they should be made to put labels on everything they produce or sell.

My personal view is that we should just put a ban on all GMO, GE foods, plants and seeds. So what is one to do? First off, let the folks in high government know your feelings, let your grocery stores realize you don't like being sold products that could cause health problems.

One should also be trying to grow their own when and wherever possible. Even if you rent a spot of ground and go from there. Container plantings just to mention one is becoming more popular and a great way to get your fresh herbs and a few veggies onto your plates.

The biggest thing you can do is to save your seeds from the original plants of years ago. Dry them and store in a cool, dry place for future use. If not for you, then for someone else that does grow their own. Give the seeds to those folks and just ask for a few fresh vegetables for your contribution.

Don't believe that these seeds will only last for a year or so if stored, as that is wrong. I have had seeds that have been saved for over twenty years and once planted flourished. Grey Wolf had seeds dating back over 60 years and planted some with great success. Nature is fantastic, almost magical, she is patient and always there to help when needed. (In her natural state that is.)

There is one thing you should know. My research shows that the plants that they are playing with regarding modification are now starting to become resistant to these chemicals, growing stronger, and given time I believe they will surely take their revenge on us. It's beginning to happen now. Plants that you can't kill with pesticides, insects that are deformed, stronger and taking control of their destiny.

If we keep on tampering with Nature, trying to alter her lifestyle, we inevitably will suffer significantly in the coming years. The powers today have to learn that they can't control Nature, nor should they. Another thing these GMO folks are saying is that if they don't do this, the world will run out of food. I believe this is the furthest thing from the truth.

There is proven evidence now that organically grown produce, non-GMO, can be grown in amounts to sustain any number of people. In other words, "we can feed the world without GMO." I will say this, at the beginning using the GMO grown seeds there is a substantial increase in productivity, but only in the beginning. It is all downhill from there. It seems to me that money takes preference over common sense.

For years, I have spoken at different events and functions on medicinal plants and things. I used to talk to the powers that be, but it was to no avail. Some have asked why I don't continue to talk to these powers that be and I say this. "They would hear my words alright, but the trouble is they wouldn't know what they meant." Oh, they would pat their soft hands together with applause at the end of my talk, but it would all be for nothing.

Truth be known, the ordinary person can't tell them anything. You say good morning to one, and they will look out the window to see. So, I just gave up trying to deal with them. I now try to deal with the average person or woman and each day spread the word of what Nature has to offer. Saves a lot of headaches.

When sick the darkest road is where one starts to recover.

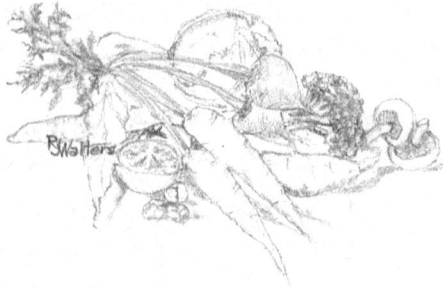

Vitamins

When it comes to vitamins these days, the store shelves are packed full. They come in all shapes, sizes and colours. They have pictures of all sorts that do their utmost to promote good health. They assure you with write-ups that say theirs is the best.

Now comes my feelings on the subject. I believe that the best way to enrich your body with what is needed in the vitamin department is to eat the foods that contain them. If you lack vitamins, you lack nutrition. There is no magic pill substitute for a proper healthy diet.

There is one vitamin today though that is lacking in a lot of peoples' bodies, that being Vitamin B-12. This vitamin plays a significant role in how one performs throughout the day. Lacking B-12 can cause nauseousness, headaches, tiredness, flu-like symptoms; the list goes on and on.

All my research says it can only be found naturally in animal foods, like meat, fish, some cheese and eggs. So for those on a vegetarian diet, it would have to be gained elsewhere, and that would have to be from a boughten source.

Cyanocobalamin is the most common type of vitamin B-12 added to a pill. Trouble is it is absorbed quite poorly. It's cheaper yes, but not as good as Methylcobalamin. It is my opinion that Methylcobalamin is a much better choice, as it is absorbed a lot better.

Its absorption is improved even more when held in the mouth and allowed to dissolve into the tissues of the mouth, instead of just swallowing it the standard way you would any other pill. Methylcobalamin in a lozenge is what I would recommend if you are in need.

Ruth's Recipes: Enjoy!

Balsamic Vinaigrette

Ingredients	Steps to cook
2 cloves (minced garlic)	Mix well in mason jar and refrigerate.
1 tbs graded Parmesan cheese	
½ tsp salt	
½ tsp pepper	
2/3 cup extra virgin olive oil	
1/3 cup aged balsamic vinegar	

Note: Great tasting dressing!

Oatmeal Raisin or Chocolate chunk Cookies

Ingredients	Steps to cook
¼ cup real butter	Preheat oven to 350 F
¼ cup organic virgin cold pressed coconut oil	Cream butter, oil and sugar. Add vanilla and eggs and blend well. Stir in oats, flour, baking powder, cinnamon and salt. Mix well. Stir in raisins or chocolate chunks.
2 cups organic coconut palm sugar	
2 tsp pure vanilla	
2 free-range organic eggs	
3 cups organic quick oats	Drop by tablespoon onto greased cookie sheet. Flatten with fork and bake for 10 minutes. Cool on rack. Makes 3 dozen delicious cookies!
1 tsp baking powder	
1 ½ cups unbleached flour or (whole wheat flour) would be okay too	
1 tsp organic cinnamon	
½ tsp. Sea salt	Variations for this recipe are numerous...You could add nuts and dried cranberries for a switch. Try out your own favourite combinations.
½ cup raisins or 70% cocoa chocolate chunks	

Note: We get a chocolate bar with 70% cocoa and break it into chunks for the chips, or you could just add cocoa to the dough along with the flour, and it will add the chocolate and no more added sugar!

Our Favourite Salad

Ingredients	Steps to cook
1 bunch organic romaine lettuce	Fill a sink with cold water add 1 cap of organic apple cider vinegar. Place vegetables in water and soak for 15 minutes. Then rinse in cold water.
½ cup organic baby spinach	
4 large leaves organic kale	
1 medium organic carrot (grated)	In a large glass bowl add the next ingredients.
1 organic broccoli tops	Chop lettuce, spinach, kale, and broccoli in fine shreds.
10 organic seedless grapes (dark)	
1 small handful raw sunflower seeds	Chop broccoli tops fine as well.
1 handful Thompson's raisins	Peel, and grate carrots on top of the lettuce and broccoli mix.
	Cut up grapes in half or quarters depending on the size. Toss on top of carrots. Then add sunflower seeds and raisins.

Note: This is a great salad combination. Packed full of nutrients for a balanced diet. Just add the Balsamic vinaigrette and you're all set. Everyone that has tried this salad has loved it.

Creamy Chicken and Cauliflower Casserole

Ingredients	Steps to cook
1 head of organic cauliflower	Wash and soak cauliflower in cold water with a cap of apple cider vinegar for 15 minutes. Rinse and cut into bit size pieces. Cook cauliflower and strain...keeping liquid for sauce.
½ cup cooked chicken breast chunks (free ranged & antibiotic free)	
2 tbs real butter	Cream sauce;
2 tbs unbleached flour	In a small sauce pan mix butter and flour together and heat on medium, heat. Slowly add the cauliflower water to the flour mixture to make a nice cream sauce. Now add the garlic and Parmesan cheese. Stir and heat through adding more water if necessary. Now add the chucks of chicken and the salt and pepper to taste and any other spices if you wish. Heat till well mixed and heated through.

Pour the cream sauce over the cauliflower. Gently stir. Then serve. |
¼ cup Parmesan cheese (organic)	
1 clove crushed garlic	
Sea salt and fresh ground pepper to taste	

Broccoli Potato Soup

Ingredients	Steps to cook
2 broccoli tops and stems	Wash broccoli and soak in organic apple cider vinegar for 15 minutes. Then rinse in cold water.
4 medium red potatoes	
Sea salt and pepper to taste	
1 tbs real butter	While that is soaking, peel and wash the potatoes. Cut potatoes in small bite size pieces. In a large pot cook potatoes till done.
	Chop the broccoli tops in bite size pieces. Grate the upper part of the stock to about 3-4 inches down. Add to potato pot.
	Cook until broccoli is done. With a potato masher mash everything together and add butter and salt and pepper to taste.
	Very simple recipe and so good for you.

Easy Dijon Roasted Potatoes

Ingredients	Steps to cook
1 ½ lbs medium red potatoes	Preheat oven to 425 F
1/3 cup organic virgin coconut oil (melted)	Wash, and cut potatoes into 8ths or mini potatoes halved. Put into a large bowl.
¼ cup Dijon mustard	
1 tbs dried oregano, basil, or rosemary leaves	
Sea salt and pepper to taste	Combine remaining ingredients together and drizzle over potatoes to coat.
	Place potatoes on a baking sheet and bake for 10 minutes then turn and bake another 10 minutes.
	Delicious !

Crumb Muffins

Ingredients	Steps to cook
2 cups unbleached flour	Preheat oven 350 F
1 ½ tsp baking powder	Blend ingredients together and reserve ¼ for topping.
1 tsp baking soda	
¼ tsp sea salt	Add : milk, egg, oil, apple sauce and vanilla in to ¾ of the top ingredients. Mix just until blended. Grease muffin tins and fill to a little over ½ full and sprinkle the toppings on each one.
¾ cup real butter	
½ cup organic coconut palm sugar	
Reserve ¼ of the top ingredients	
½ cup milk	
1 egg (free ranged)	Bake for approx. 25 minutes or until toothpick comes out clean.
½ cup melted organic virgin cold pressed coconut oil	
½ cup organic coconut palm sugar	
½ cup organic apple sauce	Great muffins for any occasion!
1 teaspoon pure vanilla	

Microwave Ovens

Today I would say that most homes have a microwave sitting on the counter in the kitchen. Are they safe to cook our food in?

Well, if you searched you would find all kinds of people, scientists, even chefs saying that they are perfectly safe, that it doesn't take anything away from our food.

On the other hand, there are just as many saying the microwave is unsafe, it releases radiation, it doesn't cook all the food all the way through and the biggie it destroys nutrients.

I am not about to tell you that either one of these explanations is right or wrong. I will tell you this.

We used to have a microwave and used it quite regularly. But a funny thing happened after using it for a while. The food started to lose its flavour. We also noticed that some our vegetables when cooked in the microwave lost a lot of their nutrients. More so in some than others. Don't get me wrong here; I know any cooking causes a loss of nutrients. My wife says our foods cooked without the microwave tastes much better, and I have to agree.

The reason we eliminated it from our lifestyle was, that simply put, there isn't enough information proving it is safe to use for cooking.

Do we miss it? My wife says not a bit. Instead, we now have a small toaster oven sitting in the microwaves spot for the small meals. The large meals are cooked in our conventional stove.

She says it doesn't take any more work or time using our old oven or toaster oven to cook with.

My opinion is this: For now I think it would be in our best interest health wise to put it aside and go back to our standard way of cooking.

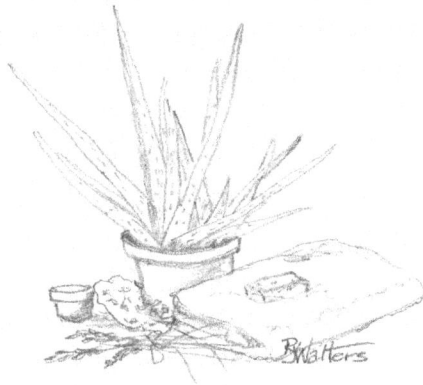

Body & Skin Care

For most the body and skin doesn't enter into the picture very often when trying to stay healthy.

What should be remembered is that what goes on your body is every bit as important as what goes into your body.

Walking through a drug store or supermarket there are literally thousands of items for one to use on their body. Most are loaded with all kinds of ingredients that I believe to be inappropriate to a person's health or well-being. Not to forget what they do to Nature too.

Reason I say this, is that all the chemicals that are put on the body at some times are eventually washed off. Where do these chemicals go? Down the drain heading towards Nature.

If you don't know the meaning of a word under ingredients, why would you put it in or on your body? Always amazes me that a lot of people use these items without giving them recognition.

So what is one to use or do? To start things off let's take a person's hair. For most, store-boughten shampoo is the item of choice. Most of these I believe aren't good.

Hair is on the head. The head is only a smidgen thick if that, till we get to the brain. We then pour all kinds of chemicals onto the hair. Shouldn't that be telling us something? If not I believe it should, as these chemicals have the ability to penetrate and do all kinds of things to someone's hair and skin. In theory, they then have the ability to go through your skin and into our brain. Not a good thing to happen, but it is a good thing to know.

Today the manufacturers of these products are telling us they are perfectly safe to use. But are they? I believe not. So what can you use on your hair?

I have found that baking soda is about the safest thing one can use. It not only cleans your hair but promotes good hair health. In doing so, your hair looks natural, clean and fresh all day long.

What my wife and I do, we take a good brand of baking soda. Pour enough into a thick small glass jar. Now fill the rest with water, swirl it around a bit and pour over your hair. (After you get it good and wet of course.) It is self-regulated. What gets mixed is what you need for each wash. The rest stays in the jar. Nothing can be simpler.

The thing that you have to get past is the lather, as there is none. People think the more lather, the better your hair will look. That isn't the case.

Once you get your hair all washed using baking soda what do you use for a soft or dry scalp? Well here again my wife and I came up with the solution. Go out and buy yourself some organic apple cider vinegar. Take another jar and mix it 50-50. Half vinegar, half water.

When you have finished washing your hair with the baking soda, rinse thoroughly. Now pour the apple cider vinegar on your hair and work in. Finally, rinse with fresh water, and you're finished! Your hair will become soft and will shine like Nature intended it to. No more harsh chemicals are entering your body.

Now you've got your hair and scalp looked after and looking good what can one use for a body wash? For your body, we recommend Kiss My Face Soap. There are probably others if you seek them out.

Next, I would like to comment on how to dry the skin after having had a bath or shower. Here again, we have been told to pat dry our skin. (Whatever you do don't rub vigorously.) Let's think about that for a second.

If a person gently pats dry, all your old dead skin is going to stay where it is and accumulate. But if you use a bit of muscle when drying, what is left on your skin will be removed. Doesn't that make sense?

I have found that by leaving this dead skin on your body, it can lead to all kinds of rashes and skin problems. For two years my body produced a rash after showering. Since I changed back to my old ways of drying, all outbreaks ceased to exist.

So when you get out of the tub, get to work and dry yourself like you're supposed to. Put some effort into that towel, and your body will thank you for it.

I also believe that most of the water we are washing our body and clothes with today isn't the best either. They say they are making it safer for us by adding chemicals. They have laws that force us to use them.

With all the chlorine and fluoride that is added to our water supply today, my conclusion is that they are causing more unhealthy bodies than they are protecting.

So what can you do to protect yourself, from those that are supposed to be protecting you? There are filters today that you can now fasten to your shower, instead of the regular shower heads. These new shower heads filter out the chlorine and fluoride before it gets to your body. I recommend these for those that live in the city or anywhere that these chemicals are being added.

Doesn't take a rocket scientist to know that if you dump poison on your body or put poison in your body, you are going to have an unhealthy body. Right?

I have some space left here. So think about this. You go to your tap; you take a glass of water with all these chemicals that they say are safe. These chemicals kill all bacteria. So the water goes into your stomach.

What happens? Well, all the bacteria good and bad in your stomach is killed. Isn't it any wonder why so many are getting sick? As our bodies need bacteria for us to live.

If we have to drink this water, we should make it a mission to replace the good bacteria daily.

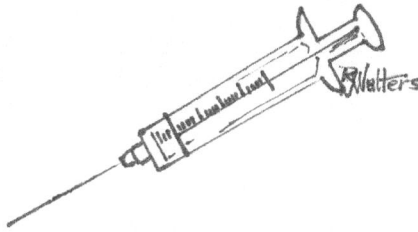

Vaccines

Here is a topic that is very controversial. Over the years I have given this topic a lot of my time researching and watching folks that have received these vaccinations like the flu shots and others.

What I believe is that vaccines override the body's immune system, which in turn depletes the body's defence against all kinds of bacteria, toxins and many other harmful things. The immune system then stops most diseases from getting past our entry points right off the bat, which is, the nose, mouth, digestive tract or other bodily points of entry. If all these fails, which sometimes happens, then the immune system being quite intelligent, doesn't just quit, it jumps into high gear, adapts to what is taking place and goes to work fighting the culprits.

When it comes to vaccines that are injected into the body, I believe it bypasses the first line of defences, which throws the body into disarray. This isn't natural and is totally out-of-order. The body then generates a temporary and incomplete immunity. With a natural exposure, the body corrects the problem, and you become immune to these diseases for a lifetime in most cases. My theory is that vaccinated individuals will never develop lifelong immunity, and will continually have to receive booster shots as protection.

So what is one to do after taking all these flu shots and different vaccinations and wants to get back on track? Well, fortunately, Mother Nature like all good mothers, is there to help us out. Eating right is the first step with the intake of lots of fresh vegetables mostly raw, along with fresh organic fruit. That will bring us the vitamin C along with lots of other good things that are needed.

Second is vitamin D from the sun. I can't stress enough about how vital the sun is, in keeping us healthy. Most folks are not getting a tenth of what is needed and need to expose their skin to the sunshine a little at a time every day.

The third is water. As I mentioned earlier, fresh water is essential, as it enables the body to perform with perfection, along with keeping us safe from all kinds of diseases. Let me refresh one last time. Freshwater, not water laden down with things like chlorine, fluoride or other chemicals.

My son Karl has his views on the subject with saying this: "You just have to look at the 3rd world countries that don't have the vaccines to see the advantages we have. Nothing is perfect, but the millions of lives saved by them is a good reason to use them. We forget how lucky we are over here. The fact that we can survive some of the most dangerous bugs in the world is a miracle."

My wife has concerns, here is what she has to say: "I have concerns of what chemicals they put into the vaccines that could harm us; along with unnecessary vaccinations for things that our immune system can fight off on its own."

My friend Dr. Graham Wood has his views. Here is what he believes. "I believe that on the whole, vaccines are good and have saved many millions of people on the planet from disability and untimely death. Ultimately, one must decide for themselves on the best course of action to be taken and take responsibility for his or her health."

So there you go. Everyone at this time has concerns, but overall things are leaning towards them as a good thing. Lastly,

I would say this. "Wouldn't it be great if we could get the doctors, scientists, pharmaceutical, chemists, researchers, naturalists like myself working together with Nature for the betterment of all mankind?"

The body is an amazing piece of equipment. If not poisoned, overworked and given the right nutrients, it will host this energy of life for many years.

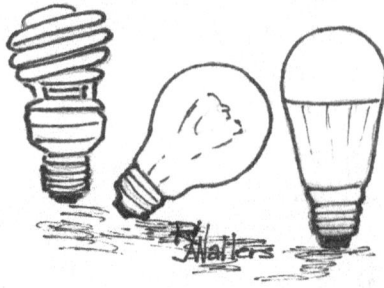

Light & Light Bulbs

Here is an interesting item that I feel is important to one's health. Today many folks are working in an inside environment, hardly ever getting outside to enjoy what Nature has provided for us free of charge. Sunshine, fresh air and plants.

So what do the powers-that-be subscribe to those that can't get outside for a few minutes each day? Well first off I think folks should make time and get outside no matter what.

What has happened here is that we rely on light bulbs to brighten up our lives. In saying this, all light bulbs are not equal, or for that matter good for you. For most of our lives we have been subjected to the old incandescent filament bulbs which in my eyes other than being a bit expensive to use was and still is about the healthiest lighting there is.

Things though have changed. As here again our powers-that-be have implemented into our lives new light bulbs, supposedly better for us, which by the way was never brought out in the open for the public to vote on.

These bulbs are called fluorescent light (CFL) bulbs. Drop and break one, and you'll have to evacuate the room quickly or breathe in mercury vapour which resides inside every bulb. The other bulb that is making headway nowadays is the LED bulb. Good bulbs in most instances, but not without some reservations which one should keep in mind. No one knows what the long-term effects of these new bulbs are going to cause.

My wife and I did switch all the bulbs in our home over to the LED, and I have to admit they sure saved us some money on our hydro bill each month. Changing all the bulbs in your house isn't cheap, but the prices of the bulbs are slowly edging lower.

The best source of light though comes naturally from our sun. Nothing is healthier for you than sunlight. I can't stress enough on how important it is for a person to get outside every day, exposing their skin to the rays of the sun.

One great way to bring the sunshine into your body is to look up at the sun with your eyes closed. Things will become red. Just hold that place for a couple of minutes and let the energy absorb through. You will be surprised how good your body performs for the rest of the day.

Today they tell folks to wear light long sleeve shirts and pants. Don't go outside without sun-blockers and stay out of the sun as much as possible. I believe all the above to be wrong and misguided information.

My Grandmother said that come spring we should start going out into the sunshine at short intervals, increasing our time in the sun each day. In doing this, along with eating good healthy food, our skin would become accustomed to the hot temperatures and the rays of the sun all summer long.

Another item that helps to deal with sunlight would be water. I can't stress enough the benefits one receives from drinking water. Everyone should drink at the least, eight glasses a day.

I believe that the reason folks burn in the sunlight is an unhealthy diet and lifestyle. Changing these things, I think one's health will improve drastically, and exposure towards the sun will then bring great rewards.

One other vegetable that helps with the body's exposure to the sun is the wild leeks. No other plant can compare to the goodness found in leeks. I should mention here that if wild leeks aren't available, an organic variety is also quite good. Just that wild leeks have in them all that Mother Nature can give you first hand.

Leeks I have found have a compound in them that darkens the texture of the skin. In doing so, this stops any harmful effects of overexposure to the sun.

The ultraviolet rays of the sun are capable of killing bacteria, viruses, fungi, yeasts, moulds, and mites. Getting out into the sun is an excellent treatment for many skin diseases, such as diaper rash, athlete's foot fungus, psoriasis, acne and boils.

My wife and I hang our sheets, towels and pillowcases in the sun on the clothes-line, as the sun kills germs quickly and makes for a pleasant fresh scent. Furthermore research also has indicated that sunlight increases pain tolerance and can bring natural body oils to the surface of the skin; which keeps the skin beautiful and smooth. The choice is yours.

Understanding Nature is the solution.

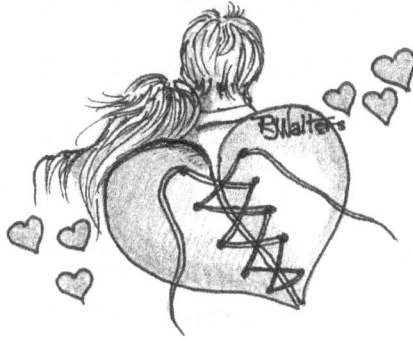

Love & Beauty

Here is a topic that most shy away from, but with my lovely wife suggesting that it would be a great asset to the book, I will do my best to enlighten you with the information that I have gathered from my friend Grey Wolf. It would be best explained by saying that people have a general desire to belong and to love which is usually satisfied within an intimate relationship. These relationships involve feelings of liking or loving one or more people and romance and physical or sexual attraction and sexual relations or emotional and personal support between each other. Intimate relationships allow a social network for people to form strong emotional attachments.

So for those that want that sparkle in their eye, here is Grey Wolf's secrets from years of experimentation. The first being, of course, lavender. There is no better around that is so easily found and works so well in the bringing together of a man and woman. The first recipe is 4 tsp dried lavender, 1 tsp pine bark, 1 tsp thyme, 1 tsp mint, 1 tsp rosemary, 1 tsp clove, and 1/2 tsp cinnamon. You can make it as an infusion and spray around the bedroom or on pillows and sheets. Or you can make it as an oil and use with a massage or a tincture used as you would any other perfume or shaving lotion. Lavender works well all on its own too.

When it comes to being fertile, you should wear green as the colour green is what the mind craves when in this state. 4 tsp mint leaves, 1 tsp pine bark, 3 tsp Vervain leaves—which you can go online and find the seeds to plant in your gardens4 tsp lavender, 2 slices of cucumber, 2 tsp hazelnuts, and 3 tsp sunflower petals. Vervain works quite well all on its own and grows well in North America. Make it as a tincture and rub on wrists twice a day and behind the ears. You can also make an infusion and drink one cup a day or you can use a combination of both.

One should wear either pink or red when looking for love. 4 tsp lavender leaves and flowers, 3 tsp peppermint leaves, 2 tsp lemon juice from rinds, 2 tsp apricot juice (fresh apricot is best), 1 tsp rosemary, 1 tsp basil, 1 tbs rose petals, and 1 tsp coriander. All are readily available in North America. Make an infusion and both you and your partner enjoy one or two cups a day. It can draw the person of your dreams into your life when applied to your neck using a tincture mixture. Grey Wolf said it was quite potent and to make sure this is the route you want to take before using.

The colour of choice to create passion is red and no other shade will do. 2 tsp vanilla, 4 sliced pieces of ginger whether dried or fresh, 2 tsp rosemary, 2 tsp mint leaves, 3 tbs avocado juice, 3 tsp hibiscus petals or leaves—calendula petals will also work—and 1 tsp clove. Make an infusion from the ingredients and apply as a mist covering your body and clothing that you are wearing at the time of intimacy. It can also be used as a mist throughout the bedroom or your place of choice.

For beauty, one should wear light blue or pink. 1 tsp Chaga ground to a powder, 2 tsp ginger root ground to a powder, 1 tsp jasmine, 4 tsp lavender leaves, 4 tbs avocado juice, 1 tsp catnip, and 1 tsp ginseng if available. A substitute would be one extra tsp of lavender. 2 tsp moss (Old-man's-beard) found here in

Northern Ontario which hangs from a lot of the trees in and around wet areas. Add 2 tsp fennel. Mix all together and make an infusion that can be sprayed on your body after bathing or made as an oil and applied to areas in need. Always test on the wrist first to make sure you're not allergic as with any potion made from Nature. It is also perfect for varicose veins.

For happiness, colours to wear are pink, blue, or yellow. 1 tsp lavender, 1 tsp sweet-pea juice (optional), 1 ½ tsp mint leaves, 1 ½ tsp catnip, 2 tsp apple blossoms, and 1 tsp St. John's wort or lemon balm if unavailable. Now make a fusion tea. One cup before breakfast makes for a great day. Beyond what most think is essential, happiness is what is most often missing. When you replace happiness in one's life, a person feels more whole and alive and self-sufficient and yet a part of the world.

Grey Wolf said to grind up a half a cup of raw organic pumpkin seeds and pour over your cereal in the mornings. You will have sexual sensations enter your body within two days. It is also very good for prostatitis in men, not to forget hundreds of other benefits that come along with eating these seeds. Always buy raw organic in seed form and grind them up yourself.

Here are a couple of items that if mixed together will give a man and woman more sensations than any other. It has been a well-kept secret for years according to Grey Wolf, only to be given out when all else fails. Whatever the reason, here it is for you to use. In saying this, I would hope that you use it sparingly and only when necessary as too much of a good thing isn't always best. Pine tree sap mixed with wild leeks.

Chew as you would a piece of gum and then swallow when you're tired of chewing. Grey Wolf said it's a super potent aphrodisiac which helps immensely with those who have impotence. These two items are perfect for those who have prostatitis. Grey Wolf with his ending remarks on the subject said, "If love still fades, that person was never yours anyway."

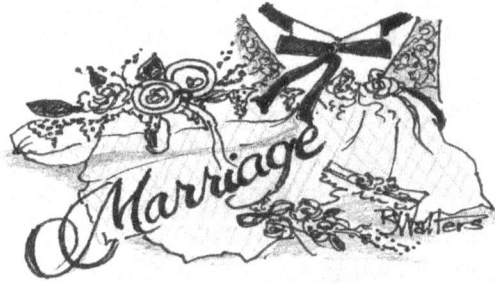

Marriage

What is a marriage?

So many folks I have found take up marriage thinking it is something that just comes naturally.

My wife and I have been married for 45 years at the writing of this book. How was this accomplished? To start off, the reason you are getting married is that you both love each other, or it should be.

At the beginning though what usually happens is that you both take to enjoying the fruits of the land so to speak. Like being lovers, enjoying each other's bodies and company. Nothing it seems at this moment in life can be better. Then the young ones make an appearance into your lives. This is another beautiful thing to happen, but in saying that, children don't come without bringing along some added challenges that some folks just can't handle.

Life becomes harder, more complicated to some. Grey Wolf said the next part had been handed down for years throughout his people.

When you enter marriage what really should happen is that you marry three people.

1-Your lover
2-A friend
3-A brother or sister

To be the best wife and husband, is you need to be:

1-A lover
2-A friend
3-A brother or sister

The way it works correctly is to apply all three at the right time when needed.

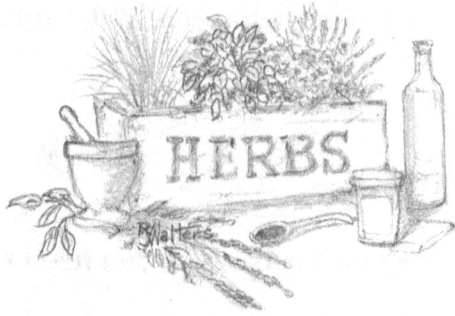

Herbs & Their Uses

Nature has provided everything we need to stay healthy if we only take the time to look. The following list are the herbs and plants that my wife and I rely on every day. They are the same ones Grey Wolf used to help folks for many years.

Think of these as the tools for your body's maintenance. Some you can find in your spice rack, and others you can grow in your own garden. Each one has a purpose.

Balm

Also known as lemon balm or sweet balm. Using the green leaves and flowers, it is a natural benefit to those that have a problem with perspiration; it will also bring boils to a head and is useful for insect stings and toothache, as well as flatulence and digestion.

Basil

This is the same basil that you use in cooking. You can make a tea from the dried herb to treat nausea. It works almost immediately for most.

Holy Basil

It is said that it increases a sense of well-being, helps the immune system, and prevents disease. It also can help with memory loss, fevers, coughs, sore throats, bites, cuts, and scrapes, along with assisting a headache. Other information says it can increase kidney function, balance emotional health, and help with acne.

Caraway Seeds
Caraway is a calming herb that will ease bloating of the stomach. It is beneficial for children. It also gives you an appetite, and because it is also an astringent, it will help laryngitis, bronchitis, and bronchial asthma.

Cayenne Pepper
Also known as capsicum, chilli or chilli pepper, hot pepper and Tabasco pepper. It is an effective treatment for pleurisy, kidney problems, skin, and colds.

Celery (Dried)
My wife and I cut and dry the celery leaves, which can be used for anti-inflammatory, anti-rheumatic, diuretic, or anti-spasmodic problems. Great for treating rheumatism, arthritis, and gout. It is also an excellent additive for soups and stews.

Chamomile
The list of benefits and treatments for chamomile are huge. A few that come to mind are insomnia, anxiety, menopausal depression, loss of appetite, diarrhea, colic, aches and pains of flu, migraine, teething, motion sickness, and inflamed skin. It is an amazing plant.

Cinnamon

Makes an excellent antiseptic and is used to treat colds. Plus, if one would take a spoonful of honey along with a spoonful of cinnamon mixed in with a cup of hot water every morning, it would help immensely with those that have high blood pressure. One of my wife's most favourite recipes—she is living proof.

Coriander
All parts of the plant are edible, but the fresh leaves and the dried seeds are the parts most used in cooking. Excellent for stomach trouble, prostate, and any urinary ailments. Can be found in most grocery stores in the herb and spice department.

Dill
Here is one that is very readily available but hardly anyone uses it, as most don't know its health benefits. It is the seeds that are used. An excellent remedy for bloating and colic, along with helping to soothe the nerves. Also, very good when making pickles.

Fennel
My wife and I use the seeds. Excellent for those that have put on a bit too much weight, because it helps take away the appetite. They help with indigestion when uric acid is the problem, and they are perfect for an acidic gassy stomach, gout, and colic in the young. It has a taste of licorice.

Fenugreek
Fenugreek seeds are excellent in the treatment of swellings, fever, blood poison prevention, and as a tea for a sore throat. Pleasant tasting herb found in the spice aisle at most grocery stores.

Flaxseed

Flaxseed has been used for years in treating a sore throat and mucous membranes. It is also excellent for mental depression and tends to help one's memory. It also can help those that are constipated along with other stomach disorders. We are never without them in our home. My wife buys only golden brown organic and grinds to our liking. We don't recommend you buy the powder, as ground flax tends to go bad quite quickly.

Garlic
Garlic stimulates the activity of the digestive organs. It has proven useful in treating asthma and whooping cough. It is also valuable in intestinal infections and very useful in reducing high blood pressure. I believe that garlic meets any health issues head-on.

Marjoram
Beneficial for the treatment of nervous disorders, helps digestion, and is used in numerous food recipes. My wife swears that it gives things flavour that had none at all.

Parsley
Parsley is rich in vitamin B and potassium. It is an excellent water pill and one of the best herbs for the gallbladder as it helps in the elimination of gallstones. Grey Wolf said he helped hundreds of folks rid themselves of unwanted gallstones by utilizing this herb.

Peppermint
Peppermint combats gas, along with being used to relieve colic, nausea, and the feeling of being sick. It's the kind of herb that should be carried around when travelling.

Psyllium

Psyllium is an excellent colon cleanser; it cleans out stored-up pockets on the colon. It also helps those being poisoned by toxic substances produced by the body.

Rosemary
Rosemary works excellently as a circulatory and nerve stimulant. It also has a calming effect on the stomach and helps those with headaches or depression.

Saffron
Saffron helps people with arthritis get rid of the uric acid which holds the calcium deposited in the joints. It can help in the reduction of lactic acid build-up and is very good for measles, skin, scarlet fever, and sweat. Not the cheapest herb, but worth every penny.

Sage
Sage makes a great tea to gargle with for an ulcerated throat or mouth. It also stops bleeding of wounds and cleans old ulcers and sores. (Note: Grey Wolf said that people with epilepsy should stay away from sage at all costs, as it can cause fits for some.)

Thyme
Thyme has a high content of oil. It is exceptionally good for coughs, throat, and asthma. It also can be used externally on infected wounds.

Turmeric
Turmeric has impressive healing powers. Research shows it can decrease certain types of tumours. I have used turmeric for years with my dandelion treatment for cancer. It is an anti-inflammatory and antioxidant which can help those suffering from osteoarthritis and rheumatoid arthritis.

Oatmeal
There is nothing better than a bowl of oatmeal porridge for lowering your blood pressure. Eat one bowl every day, without sugar. Add natural fruits instead.

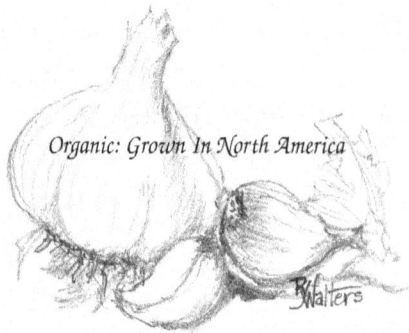

Organic: Grown In North America

Garlic

Garlic is one vegetable that triumphs over all others. For years, I have grown garlic of all kinds, and there isn't a day that goes by that my wife doesn't add it to one of our meals.

Garlic is the immune system's best friend. My research says that fresh garlic has proven to help destroy viral infections such as measles, mumps, chicken pox, herpes simplex 1 and 2, herpes zoster and many types of bacterial illnesses including streptococcus, diarrhea, tuberculosis, and tetanus.

It is also said to be very good for helping those with high blood pressure and heart disease and is a great strength builder. Raw garlic can be eaten at the first sign of a cold or flu to ward off the illness or to lessen the symptoms. One should remember though that raw garlic is an emetic, so go slowly and stop eating if nauseousness occurs.

For other infections, garlic can be used externally as well as internally. It is quite strong and could burn sensitive areas. I have gone as far as taking a raw piece of garlic and holding it on the infected area. It did sting some, but within two days the infection and pain were gone.

Grey Wolf said that if you were having some awful luck with sickness or money, a person would merely hang a piece of garlic over the doorway. No bad luck would then be allowed to enter. Something that you could try if you had a mind to. He did have some non-standard ideas now and then.

Garlic is well-known for its strong disagreeable odour and its taste which is stronger than onions. It is said that the scent of garlic or peppermint can improve reasoning, problem-solving, concept formation, judgment, attention span, and even memory.

My wife and I love it, and I usually have a raw clove every other night just before supper. Put it together with a piece of home-made bread, and you're in for a great treat and so good for you too.

A person has to understand that the garlic from the store could have been sprayed with a hormone, which prevents it from sprouting. Try to seek out some garlic that has been grown local organically if you plan on planting your own. Give it a try; you'll be surprised at how easy it is to grow!

I like to plant mine just before the ground freezes. I break the bulb apart and plant one clove root down into a hole about 2 inches deep and 3 inches apart. To make the hole for planting, I just use the handle of my hoe. Once done I cover with soil and leaves. That's it.

If you do purchase garlic from the grocery store look for these words on the label, as you're more likely to have garlic that has not been sprayed with a growth inhibitor: "organic" or "all natural". Also, the garlic that comes from countries other than North America does not have roots hanging from the bottom. Come spring you will see it shooting up and out of the ground. Sometimes even with the snow still being around.

It's sad when some can't see what stands before them.

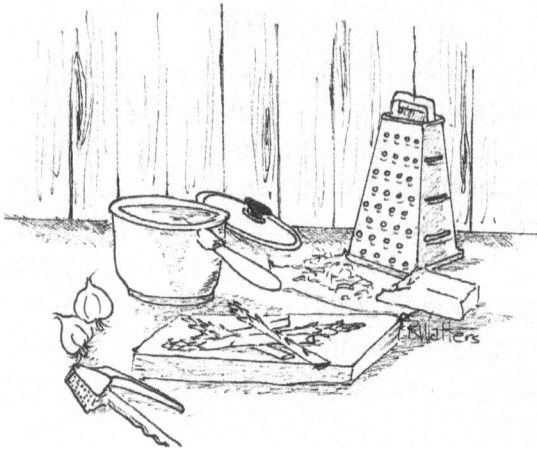

Asparagus

Asparagus is another excellent vegetable. My wife and I try to have some once a week with our meals. It is good cooked or chopped up and mixed in with a salad. Very good for you and has many medicinal properties. It is a diuretic, which means it has a substance that tends to increase the flow of urine, causing the body to get rid of excess water.

Grey Wolf said that this is a common garden vegetable which can be used either as a tea or in decoction.

My research says that asparagus tea is good for stones or gravel in the kidneys or bladder and is made by soaking the roots in hot water, but not boiling, for ½ hour then strain. Remember boiling eliminates most of all the good things in vegetables and plants.

It is also said that asparagus is very good for those with Alzheimer's or memory loss. Studies also show it is an excellent anti-inflammatory along with helping digestive problems, regulating blood sugar and has lots of anti-cancer benefits, especially leukemia.

So next time you're in the supermarket why not add a bunch or two to your shopping cart. Your body will be glad you did.

One last thing, don't be worried if your urine smells after eating asparagus, as that is a common trait of what it does going through your system.

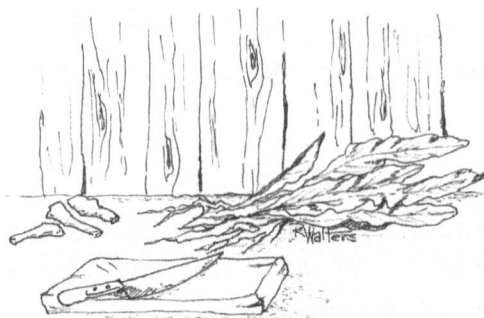

Horseradish

Horseradish is a potent stimulant. My research says it is outstanding in treating arthritis and rheumatism. Internally it can be made into a tea. Externally it can be made using oil.

Findings also say that horseradish contains antibacterial, antibiotic, and antiparasitic properties. It is also useful for the heart and as an expectorant (which means it helps clear the lungs and stimulates many body systems), and can be used to aid mild circulatory problems, digestion, and water retention. An effective daily dose of horseradish can be as little as 1 gram, which is a touch less than a teaspoon.

Back on the farm, I had a row of horseradish around twenty feet long, and after two years we had more than we could use. Eventually, we were digging it and selling it on the farmers market.

I have said this many times. Drugs do not heal, they treat symptoms. What does heal, though, is our immune system.

If you treat it well and give it proper nutrition, it can fix pretty well anything.

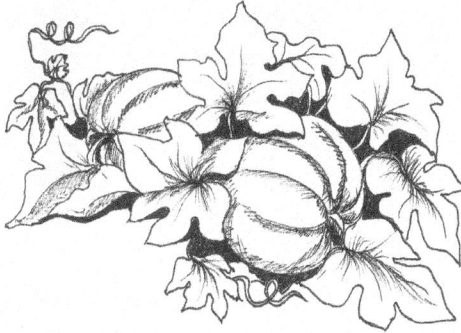

Pumpkin

This is one of my favourite vegetables, especially when made into pies. But other than the pies, it also has a lot of medicinal qualities. For those who are dealing with serious health challenges, I highly recommend you start taking the seeds—organic and raw, of course—grinding them up and eating at the minimum of a 1/4 cup a day.

The chemicals in the pumpkin seeds also cause an increase in urination which helps relieve bladder discomfort, along with supporting those who have prostatitis.

Eating raw organic pumpkin seeds is about the best remedy there is out there today for treating those with a tapeworm. Hardly heard of anymore, but there are a few that are still being bothered by this pest. For positive results one must eat only organic, raw seeds, either shelled or with shells on. Both have the power to eliminate this rascal, along with intestinal parasites as well. The best time to eat the seeds for treating tapeworms is at night before retiring.

Research says that pumpkin also acts as a sedative which induces sleep. In doing so, it can be beneficial for those struggling with mental balance and restlessness, including insomnia, agitation, and depression. Along with all that, the mighty pumpkin helps those dealing with memory loss, as it improves one's focus and makes the mind more stabilized.

Pumpkin is also used to treat boils, carbuncles, fever, measles, skin ailments, sprains, and warts. Its seeds will also help promote clarity and help the body eliminate kidney stones with the chemicals it possesses.

Now that you have a list of things that the pumpkin can help you with, there is one last item that most don't know. The flowers are delicious mixed in with salads, or one can do as I do and mix a few in with your homemade bread. Just a couple makes the bread quite tasty along with giving it a great colour.

When planting pumpkins, once the blossoms start to show themselves, I take a cotton swab and touch all the centres of the flowers, moving around the pollen from plant to plant. This helps in its propagation. With the lack of honey-bees these days, our plants need all the help they can get to produce.

Roasted pumpkin seeds recipe:

Separating the seeds from the pulp and roasting them is the best way to enjoy the health benefits of the pumpkin. Here is how my wife and I prepare them:

Clean the Seeds: Separate the seeds from the pumpkin pulp and rinse them thoroughly under cold water to remove any remaining stringy bits.

Coat: Toss the clean seeds in a small amount of butter or organic coconut oil until they are lightly coated.

Season: Sprinkle a bit of natural sea salt over the seeds to your liking.

Bake: Spread them on a baking sheet and bake at 325°F for 25 to 30 minutes.

Stir: Make sure to stir the seeds every 5 minutes to ensure they brown evenly and don't burn.

Finish: Let them cool completely before eating.

Enjoy! These make a fine, healthy snack that supports the body while tasting just like a treat.

Understanding Nature in her many forms can be of a great benefit to your health.

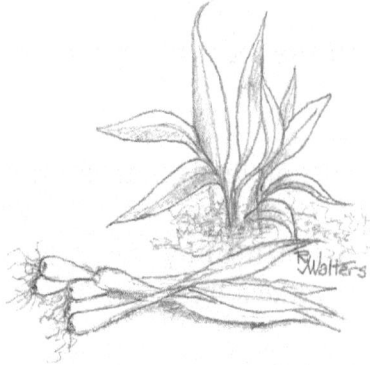

Wild Leeks

A person can never go wrong venturing out into the bush to seek out these nutritional plants come spring.

Grey Wolf used to say that the body is like water: it has to be kept moving, if not it becomes stagnant. Especially in the spring of the year after being cooped up all winter. Walking with Nature seeking out the leeks improves things quite quickly.

He also recommended that the sick eat the leaves for colds, croup, and as a spring tonic. They also help ward off allergies of summer if eaten in the spring.

I have personally seen folks with terrible allergies find relief overnight just by eating a bowl of home-made wild leek soup before retiring for the evening. My wife and I go and dig them as soon as the bulbs are large enough, usually April through May. We then dry the leaves and bulbs for soups and stews when not in season.

For those with an earache, Grey Wolf would warm the juice from the leaves or bulbs and put a couple of drops in the infected area. Works miracles he said.

Usually, wild leeks are harvested in their entirety; the plant is pulled or dug from the ground including its leaves and bulbs. All parts of the plant are edible, but the outer layer of the bulb should be disposed of as it serves as a protective layer for the bulb and isn't meant to be eaten. Won't hurt you, but hard to chew.

You should remember though when digging the leeks that once you remove a few, it opens the area for other invading plants. This happens quite rapidly and should be avoided if at all possible. We only take a few here and there, keeping in mind what will happen if we take too many. So dig a few then move to another area a few feet away. Doing so will protect your supply of wild leeks for years to come.

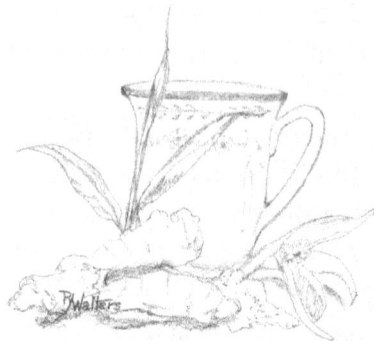

Ginger Root

For years my wife and I have used ginger roots made into a tea to help bring on a good night's sleep. It is a plant that can be used as a spice or medicinally.

My research says when made into a hot tea it can bring on sweating which in turn helps the body eliminate certain ailments, including colds and flu. Today it seems that if one gets a fever, they need to take something to bring it down. My research also says that a fever is a tool the body uses to fight infections and help one's recovery. With that in mind, a low-grade temperature might be better left alone in some cases.

Ginger, if taken too strong, can also bring on a fever-like feeling, so one has to find that happy medium. It is nice coming in on a cold day and having a hot cup of ginger tea. It warms one up in a matter of minutes.

It is said that ginger is also useful for an upset stomach, diarrhea, gas, and poor circulation. It is also a very powerful anti-inflammatory which helps those dealing with joint pains and tendinitis. Everyone should have it on hand, if for nothing else than an enjoyable drink now and then.

To enjoy it, you can dry it, then grind it up with a coffee grinder and use it in all kinds of different dishes. To make a tea, just slice off three or four pieces and place them in your tea-pot, pouring boiling water over the top. Allow it to sit for fifteen minutes and enjoy.

To correct our mistakes in life, we have to venture back to the beginning.

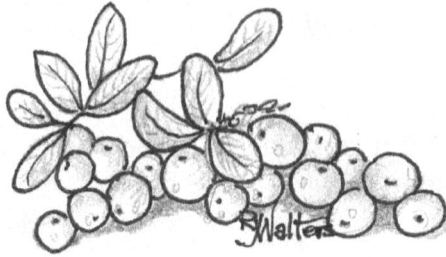

Cranberries

Cranberries for years have been used to help those with all kinds of problems. The main ones being infections in the bladder and urinary tract.

Grey Wolf's notes said that most urinary infections could be managed using nothing other than organic cranberry juice. He went on to say that even eating them crushed had a positive effect on all kinds of health issues.

The reason they work so well for urinary infections is that they possess a substance that coats the bladder and urethra, which helps prevent E. coli and other harmful bacteria from sticking to them. In turn, this allows the bacteria to be more easily eliminated through one's urine.

I have also found that drinking three or four glasses of real juice twice a week helps support the body against inflammation. I also found that if one would take a good brand of probiotics along with the cranberry juice, it helps the system recover even quicker.

Now here's the thing. Most folks today go to the grocery store and pick up a bottle of juice. Truth be known, this juice often isn't good for much. It is mostly made up of sugar and syrup along with other additives that aren't good for you. In fact, I wouldn't hesitate to say it could make a urinary infection worse instead of better because bacteria thrive on sugar.

The best way to get results is to buy either organic raw cranberries or frozen whole organic cranberries. Once you have these at home, you bring them to a boil, then let them simmer until they become soft. Do not over-boil them as that kills off the nutrients. Just put enough water to cover them. Once they are soft, you crush them up with a potato masher, double the water, and let them sit for a good half hour. You then strain and cool.

Now you have what is needed: fresh, healthy juice without chemicals or sugar. Drink one to two glasses a day until you feel better. Do not add sugar, as that will take away the benefits. It is a bit bitter, but look beyond that. You do want to be better, don't you?

Notes say that cranberry juice may help the body manage certain enzymes, which is a great asset to long-term health. Cranberries also have the capability of helping those with lung discomfort. I have come up with a remedy that I found worked well when I was dealing with a severe cough or congestion.

If you look back to how the cranberry stops bacteria from sticking to the urinary tract, that put up a flag for me. If the lungs are congested, it means the body is having a hard time clearing things out. I thought if I mixed up a batch in some steaming water and inhaled the vapours, it might stop the sticky mucus from clinging to the lungs. I tried it and it worked quite well; in a day or so, things started to clear up.

I have also used good pine shavings boiled in water and inhaled the steam, which helped with a bad sinus cold. Use one handful to three quarts of water. Make sure though you aren't on any other medication or allergic to pine.

Another thing I have found through experience is that many folks have H. pylori in the stomach. We know today that many folks with stomach ulcers have a great amount of H. pylori. There is a medical treatment consisting of proton pump inhibitors and antibiotics. It works, but it can leave the stomach in rough shape because it kills all the good bacteria too.

What is a natural alternative to support the stomach? Cranberry juice has been studied for its effect on H. pylori. My notes say it can help stop the bacteria from taking hold without killing the good bacteria. I can't prove it to be 100% true for everyone, but I think it would be worth trying.

The other is ginger root tea, or cabbage juice. My notes say that for helping the stomach recover from an ulcer, one glass of cabbage juice a day for two weeks is best. I am speaking through experience here, as I went through the ordeal of a severe ulcer myself. It is like anything else in life; one has to be willing to learn.

What we truly are, disease or famine can never destroy.

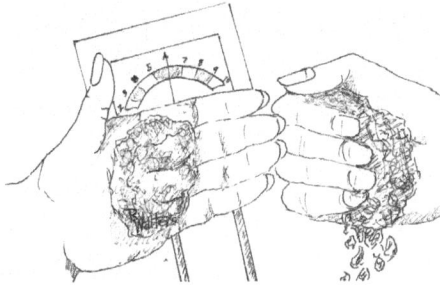

Soil

Most people never take a second look at soil when it comes to healing.

There are four basic types: clay soil, sandy soil, loam soil, and peat soil. Clay soil is the hardest to work with, but with a little ingenuity and understanding, it can produce some excellent crops. Sandy soil is easier to work with, while loam is the middle between sandy soil and clay soil. Peat soil is quite rare, containing many nutrients.

Clay in itself has fantastic healing properties. It is rich in minerals and trace elements which can be used as a mineral supplement in combination with plant extracts or herbal teas. The type of clay most used is called Bentonite clay. Minerals present in clay include calcium, chromium, copper, iron, magnesium, manganese, phosphorus, potassium, sulfur, selenium, silica, and zinc.

Clay does contain aluminum. When taken internally, because of the high silica content, the aluminum is not deposited in the body. In fact, silica helps manage aluminum and other metals that may be already in the body and carries them out. Quite interesting.

Externally, Grey Wolf used clay and water for skin irritations like blemishes, insect bites, cuts, skin itching, or burns. He would leave it on until it dried and then wash off. This, he said, produced a soothing effect on skin that is itching

93

from eczema, psoriasis, and chicken pox. I used it for shingles years ago which worked quite effectively.

Skin Poultice for Bites, burns, cuts, stings, and shingles:

For nasty problems, Grey Wolf would create a poultice by putting a thick layer of clay on the skin and applying a wet cloth over it to hold it in place. He would leave the dressing on, changing it every hour. You can buy Bentonite clay almost anywhere these days. Myself, I use our clay where we live now. It is quite plentiful after digging down a ways, and I have found it works well.

On another note, let's look at what grows in soil. Take tomatoes. In most instances today, on the outside they look delicious—appetizing, you might say. On the inside, though, some are lacking the minerals that we need to stay healthy. One primary mineral that is lacking is called selenium, which in itself can help support the body against many diseases.

One tomato, if grown in good soil, should consist of close to 57 minerals. Today we would be fortunate to get five or six. The reason this has happened is that over the years our soil has become depleted of the good things. When my father and I farmed, the old saying was: "You only get out of the soil what you put back into the soil." What has happened today is most farmers use just human-made chemicals to fertilize their crops, which is okay but not enough.

To replenish the soil, organic matter—such as horse, cow, chicken, or pig manure—is needed. It should, of course, come from free-range animals that aren't full of hormones, antibiotics, or other chemicals. Good compost is another alternative: leaves, grass-cuttings, wood ashes, along with the food you discard. It all breaks down into what is needed to replenish the soil back to a healthy state.

You know? If you look at the bottle of Heinz Ketchup, it used to say "Heinz 57." What that meant was that their tomatoes came from 57 different varieties.

My Dad said it should have indicated that there were 57 kinds of minerals in the tomatoes. An exciting thing about vegetables is that each plant has a different mineral absorption profile.

A tomato will absorb a certain number of minerals—around 57—and it will consume no more. It will only absorb the 57 that it is programmed to incorporate. It can only absorb what is made available in the soil.

Nature is amazing.

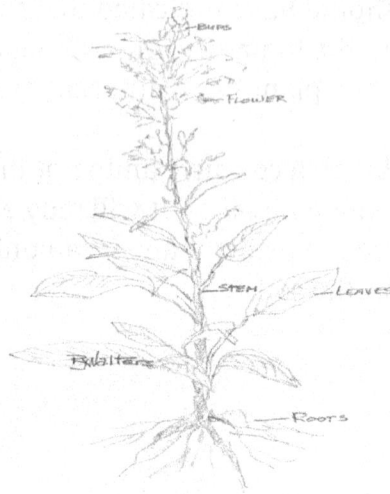

Burs

Flower

Stem — Leaves

Bulalters

Roots

Parts Of Plants

For those that would like to make medicines out of plants, I have divided them up into different parts: the roots, inner and outer bark, stems, buds, leaves, flowers, saps and pitches, fruits and seeds. Each one of these is used in different fashions to make various medicines. Each has a procedure that one must follow to get the fullest values when all is said and done.

Always make sure where you are digging or harvesting your plants that they are free of any chemicals, or any human-made items that could cause health issues. Don't get to thinking that this is going to be too much for one to comprehend as it isn't; it just consists of common sense.

Roots of plants and trees I have found contain the highest levels of nutrients in the fall and early spring. That is when I like to dig them and dry them. To better understand the harvesting of plants, it all boils down to where the plant stores most of its life-saving medicines. That being the roots for most. You should be careful though when digging the roots of plants because if you take all the roots, leaving nothing, all will be lost for future use.

Myself, when finding the plants that I want to harvest, I take a careful look around. If they are in vast quantities, I then take only the plants from the outside edge. I have always believed that the middle of the group is the old-timers. They have been around for years and deserve to carry on without people interfering with their life cycle. Truth be known, the younger ones hold just as many excellent properties as the older plants, maybe in some cases even more—especially if a person is looking for tenderness.

Annual plants are seldom used to make medicines. Perennial plants are what is used as they store all the good medicinal properties each year in their roots for the following growing season. Roots should be dug, then dried naturally leaving a bit of the soil attached. What shakes off is all that is required. The more I have worked with roots, the more I have found that the medicinal properties that are in the soil on the roots are as important as the properties that are in the root itself.

Stems of the plants are best taken once the leaves have formed on the stem itself, just before flowering.

Barks I like to harvest from trees in the fall of the year, as I have found that it doesn't cause the tree to bleed as much. In the spring of the year, if cut, it will bleed quite profoundly causing the tree some grief. If a person is in desperate need of the barks for a treatment and has no other bark on hand, then one can proceed to take what is needed. I take the inner or outer bark from the smaller branches, not touching the larger ones. It works just as well as the main bark from the trunk and is a lot easier to get at.

I take a bit of bark from different places throughout the tree, as I have found that different strengths are contained in different areas. Never strip the bark continuously around the circumference of the branch as that will kill it. I just like to take a strip off the length, leaving at the minimum of three-quarters left to carry on. This works excellent and hardly hurts the branch.

Leaves should be gathered before the flowers develop and before they start to wilt in the fall. They should only be picked after the morning dew has dried and then before the sun becomes hot, like when the sun is right overhead. If leaves are free from moisture, they dry just that much faster when brought into the house, leaving less chance of any mould forming.

Flowers are gathered just before they are fully developed as that is when the scent and properties are at their peak. When harvesting the flower, do so only after the dew has dissipated. Never wash the flowers; just shake them, and if there are any unwanted insects in them, they will fall out. If washed, they lose any good that they have in them. I have also found it best to dry flowers in the shade rather than in the sunlight or artificial heat sources.

Saps and Pitches I take either in the spring of the year or the fall. Sometimes I even take it when I see it seeping from a wound. It brings on a sad feeling when I look at the sap or pitches (pitches is like gum), as it seems they were bleeding. To humans, bleeding means pain. So when taking, I always thank the tree and give it a pat saying, "All is well, thanks."

Fruits I have found are best harvested just before they are fully ripe, especially for making elixirs and syrups for cold medicines. It seems that the acid at this time isn't as strong and makes for a better blend. Although, if you are making wine from the fruit, the riper, the better, as the riper the fruit gets, the more acid and sugar it produces. Kinda depends on what you are planning on doing with the fruit.

Seeds—make sure you pick only when dry and just before sprouting, and store in a cool, dark, dry area.

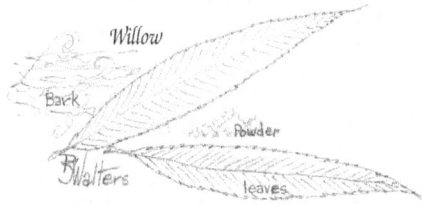

Headaches

Over the years I have seen many folks suffering from headaches. The elements around a person cause most, and each headache seems a bit different. I used to get some pretty severe headaches. After heading off to a doctor friend of mine, I found that I had some degenerated discs in the back of my neck. Problem found, but what to do?

I had a bit of therapy done where they hooked up a sling-like apparatus around your neck, pulling your head in an upward direction. I have to say it did work for a while, but in time the headaches returned. They wanted to do some surgery on my neck, but something told me that wasn't the answer. So, I did some research.

It took some time, but I found that what caused most of my headaches could be chalked up to nutrition, dehydration, and tension. Taking it one step further, I asked myself these simple questions: Have I eaten enough today? Have I had enough water to drink? Have I had a lot of caffeine, or not as much as I usually do? Is my jaw, neck, or upper back feeling tense or sore? Am I feeling nauseated, dizzy, or sensitive to light or sound?

After looking at all these things I then decided on what needed to be done to rectify the problem on my own. I found using information about what others are doing, for the most part, was useless, as everyone's headache is different. I found that individual elements can start a headache, so I eliminated them one by one over time. What amazed me was that I found all kinds of things that brought them on: computer and TV screens, fluorescent lights, loud noise, and caffeine. Coffee in some instances can help a person, as there are some chemicals in coffee that can be beneficial.

So what is one to do? I found that for most of my headaches, drinking lots of water helped immensely. Sometimes though it wasn't enough, and I found then a snack was needed, usually one with a high amount of protein like good aged cheese or nuts.

Then comes a headache that just doesn't want to go away no matter what you do. For them, I rub a bit of lavender essential oil on my temples, or put a few drops into a handkerchief and inhale. It works nine out of ten times. If all fails, I take one spoonful of willow bark and half a spoon of chamomile with a touch of lemon and make myself a tea. One cup twice a day, Grey Wolf said, should be efficient (morning and night). Unless it is eliminated sooner, don't drink any more. Only take what is needed.

The active substance in aspirin, salicylic acid, is named after the Latin name for Willow, Salix. Grey Wolf used willow bark as a painkiller for years saying it was of great help. My sources say that willow in its natural state works much better than in the pill form of today because it has all the other properties that Nature put into it. Some folks can't take aspirin as it bothers their stomach or thins their blood too much. Hope this helps, as I know how a headache can make you feel.

Only those with closed minds can be fooled.

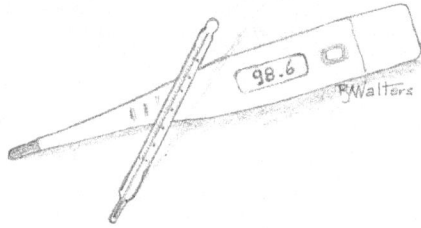

Fevers

Some see fevers as dangerous, and we should end it. I believe this isn't always correct.

My research indicates that a fever is the body's way of fighting off viruses and bacteria. I also have found through experimentation that it helps to manage stress. In some places, it has been found that a fever has been used for the treatment of some forms of cancer. With my cancer, I started inducing a fever by drinking ginger root tea before going to bed. What it did, I believe, was raise my temperature enough to help my body get on with what it should be doing. Along with that and other natural help, I have made out quite well for a good many years.

I feel that a fever is not something that we should end immediately, but there are times a temperature can become a problem. If you can stay inside and rest and the fever isn't too high, I believe it is often best to not intervene. A nice cup of chamomile and mint leaf tea, three times a day, will go a long way with your recovery.

You can also apply cold compresses to the head, neck and feet to draw the heat out of the body. Or you can dip a wash cloth in a bowl of warm water mixed with a cup of vinegar. Wring it out, and apply to the forehead. You should try to stay in a cool environment, but don't get chilled.

In saying all this, if you feel like you're going to have a seizure or feel as if you are going to pass out, or losing bodily functions, then you should contact your health provider as soon as possible. Other signs of things going wrong would be a terrible headache accompanied by a stiff neck from something like whiplash, a fall, or a bump on the head. The main thing is don't get all excited; listen to yourself, relax, and go from there.

Humour has the ability to transform people from being negative to positive.

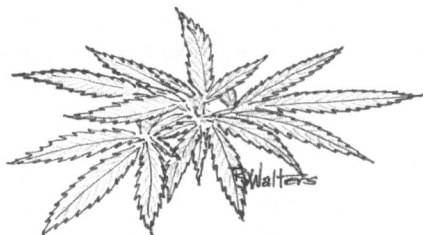

Marijuana Cannabis

When it comes to the healing power of plants, Cannabis is a heavyweight that was misunderstood for far too long. Since its legalization in Canada in 2018, the air has cleared enough for us to see the truth: this is a natural medicine, not a street drug. Unlike alcohol, which is a human-made poison that destroys the liver and the brain, marijuana grows from the earth and works with the body. I have lost friends to hard drugs and chemical overdoses, but I have never seen a person die from using a plant in its natural state.

To understand why it works, one has to realize that our bodies are actually built to receive it. We have a system inside us that responds to the chemicals in the plant, helping to balance our nerves and our pain. I have found that marijuana is a superior option for managing the deep, grinding ache that comes with cancer or aging joints.

It can be taken internally as a clean oil or applied externally as a rub. The rub is especially good because it goes right to the site of the pain—like a swollen knee or a sore back—without affecting the mind. In my view, it is a much kinder choice for the body than the harsh, toxic treatments often pushed by modern medicine. It settles the stomach, brings back the appetite, and allows a person to move through their day without being clouded by synthetic painkillers.

It is also a fine tool for the mind. It calms the nervous system and helps those struggling with the heavy weight of stress or the frustration of a sleepless night. Of course, like any medicine, you have to find your own "happy medium" and take baby steps at first. As long as we keep it natural and don't let officials start tinkering with its structure, I believe it is one of the best allies we have for a healthy, joyful life.

Where Nature hides, most never search.

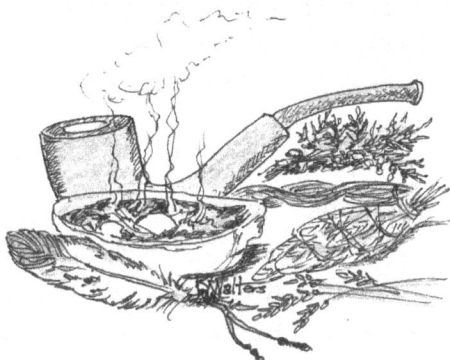

Burning Barks & Herbs

I for years have burned different herbs and barks, if for nothing else than the aroma they give off. The types I burn mostly is a combination of cedar and sage. It is not only a great way to attract the positive energy that is around us, but it is also quite healthy for you—within limits, of course. They say once a week would be sufficient.

Another one I have on hand is Chaga, which grows on the white and yellow birch trees. There is a section relating to Chaga later in this book, but it is worth mentioning here that other than the medicinal properties, it can be used to keep your smudge pots burning. The slightest touch from a flame will send it into a smouldering state which lasts for quite a spell. Natives years ago used it to carry their fires when moving from place to place.

I also enjoy burning mullein leaves and roots, dried and cut into small pieces. My notes say that the smoke can be of some help in the treatment of lung discomfort. I know on a personal note that mullein can work wonders. Years ago, I had a severe case of bronchitis. I coughed so hard and for so long that I actually ripped the muscles in my chest. It was incredibly painful, and the modern drugs the doctors gave me weren't doing a thing to stop it.

Not knowing what to do, I referred back to the old fixes I learned from my Native friends. I made a tea using the mullein leaves. Within just two cups, taken a few hours apart, my cough completely disappeared. If you try this, you must remember that mullein leaves have tiny hairs on them that can irritate the throat. You have to strain the tea very well to remove them; I always use an unbleached coffee filter to make sure it's clear.

Another plant that was smoked years ago was unprocessed tobacco. It was nothing like the tobacco of today; it didn't have a whole mess of chemical additives, which in my eyes makes modern smoking extremely dangerous. But like anything, everything should be used in moderation and not before a lot of research is done.

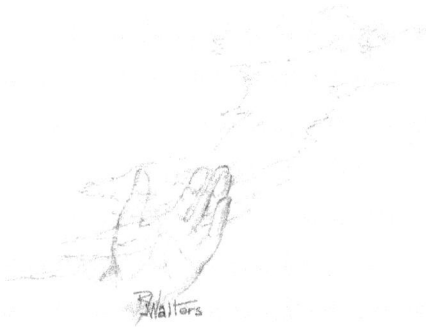

Power Of Touch

Some say there is one other viable source of healing. It is called the power of touch. It's where a gifted person can redirect the surrounding energy in such a way that it is sent into the body of need, allowing the healing to take place.

Grey Wolf said the healer sees the problem in the body through this energy, analyzes it in their mind, and then removes it—self-discarding it before it can do damage to themself. That is the trick, he said. Grey Wolf believed that only the gifted ones had such abilities.

He went on to say that it is an all-but-lost natural ability. There are a few that still have this power, but most fear it. They don't understand it, and as with anything that is misunderstood, it's usually brushed aside. He said that the gifted ones should pass on their knowledge, extinguishing the fear.

My views. Most of my life I have believed that there is a source around us more powerful than one can imagine. Not in a religious sense, but energy that seems to captivate those that choose to recognize its presence. I have concluded that recognizing this energy and utilizing it would be a great asset to those in need, be it health or just plain peace of mind.

The Unseen

This is a story taken from my collections. It is called: The Unseen. In ways, it shows the unseen-able that can occur in a person's mind without them even realizing it.

- Walking with my friend Grey Wolf wouldn't be just casual. It was—well, let me try to explain. Some things around us move so slow that the eye can't comprehend their meaning without taking the time to examine them in their entirety. Like lightning shooting down from the sky above. Does it come from above or is it an illusion?

- Cloud-to-ground lightning comes from the sky down, but the part you see comes from the ground up. So, in reality, it is both, but we only recognize the one that isn't real. I for one when young would sit for hours watching a lightning storm, mesmerized by what it was portraying. Pictures of all kinds came to mind while gazing upon its might.

- Rocks are another deceiving item, as many a time I walked right by one with Grey Wolf halting me, showing me what it contained or what it showed, as a face of some animal or human. One can get quite taken in observing such an event. Flowers are another species of particular value, with most passing them by without a second glance.

- Take the Violet. In just their leaves they show a heart shape, letting us know of the medicinal values it holds. If allowed, they could help those with heart-related concerns. By looking at a tree imagining it without its leaves, all sorts of things

108

come to view. From creatures of fantasy to reality, they are all there to enjoy if one chooses to do so.

- Clouds are quite evident in what they would like everyone to see, but here again the unseen usually gets passed by. Did you know you can even tell what the weather will be by looking at the clouds? Take mares' tails or wisps, as they trail along the sky. It is a sure sign of rain or snow within 24 hours. I even saw a bird one time with the overlap of colours showing it to be two birds instead of one. Or so it seemed.

- Then comes the unseen things like grains of sand, snowflakes, drops of water on a pond or lake, and dew on the leaves of trees or plants—each one being slightly different, invisible to the naked eye. To explain it more clearly, I would say the unseen is like an abstract put together by an artist with vision beyond recognition. Or maybe like a dream catcher that hangs from one's window, in hopes of catching what we all crave but won't say out loud for fear of being criticized. To me, the unseen allows us to see into the future, that is if we allow it to take place.

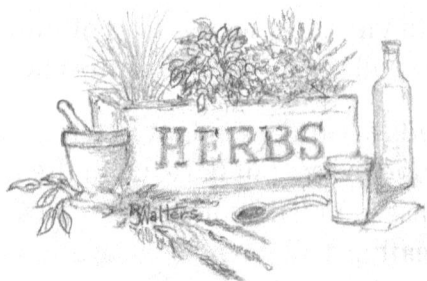

Plants Made Into Medicine

Teas & Infusions: These are made by pouring boiling water on the plant or bark and allowing it to steep for a short time until it cools, after which it is strained. Occasionally, cold water is used. Infusions are generally better than decoctions as boiling destroys the virtue of some herbs. Usually, 1 to 4 ounces of the herb should be used to a pint of boiling water.

Decoctions: A decoction is a solution made by boiling a herb or plant in water and straining while hot. Decoctions are made much like boiling coffee.

Cerates: These are ointments containing 30% beeswax to 70% lard, coconut oil, or lanolin. Cerates are used when you don't want quick-dissolving to take place. Ointments are softer, made without beeswax, using lard, coconut oil, or petroleum jelly. The medicine is mixed into the base and dissolves quickly when put on the skin.

Extracts: These are made by taking the soluble parts of the plant by allowing them to stand in water or alcohol. Fluid Extracts are made the same way but are not allowed to evaporate as much as solid extracts.

Syrups: To make a syrup, first make a strong tea (infusion) of your plant, then add sugar or a thick sweetener while hot and somewhat evaporated, then bottle.

Tinctures: These are solutions of medicinal properties in alcohol or a mixture of alcohol and water. For every 1 ounce of herb, add 2 ounces of water and 2 ounces of alcohol (I often use a good vodka). Let it stand in a bottle for 8 to 14 days in a cool place, then strain. Apple cider vinegar is a great alternative solvent; it is an antiseptic and cheaper than vodka, though it won't keep quite as long.

Fomentation: This is where you put your herbs into a bag and steep them. Wring the bag out and apply it to the affected area while hot. Grey Wolf said it was the best of the best for many an ailment. Liniments are similar but use oily substances, often mixed with plant extracts for rubbing into the skin.

The Natives also used colours to distinguish plants. A pale pink or yellow plant was often a sign it might be poisonous, while a bright violet-pink indicated medicinal plants. A sharp or dull white plant was an indication it might have power-plant properties—hallucinogenic or narcotic. It is best to go with what you know, as Nature can be cruel if not handled wisely.

How my wife and I make Herbal Salves & Balms:
Warm 1 cup of herb-infused oil in a pot over low heat.
Add 5 tablespoons of grated beeswax; stir until melted.

The Freezer Test: Dip a spoon in the mix and put it in the freezer for a minute. If it's too hard, add more oil. If too soft, add more wax.

Once right, pour into clean containers.
Add 2–3 drops of Vitamin E or essential oil per ounce just as you pour.
Let harden slowly. Keep in a cool place so they don't go rancid; they usually last about 3 months.

Poultice Preparations:

A Poultice is used to soothe, heal tissue, and draw out toxins. Mix your herbs with enough boiling water to make a thick paste. Apply as hot as possible without burning the skin. You can add coconut oil to keep it moist or wrap the paste in cheesecloth before applying. I can't stress enough how well these work in eliminating pain when prepared correctly.

Grey Wolf in his notes said:
"Disease is the result of us breaking away from Nature"

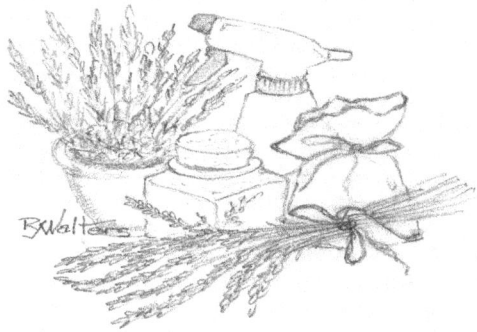

Lavender

Lavender is one of the greatest herbs known to man and produces many medicinal remedies along with just plain smelling good. First off, lavender for years has been used as an aphrodisiac. The scent of lavender, especially when combined with pumpkin pie spice, is known to be one of the most arousing aromas in the world, though it works quite well on its own too.

Let's take a look at why it's so healthy for the body and mind. It is known all over the world for being an antiseptic, antibacterial, anti-fungal, and anti-inflammatory. It can also help the body manage stress, anxiety, exhaustion, and irritability. It is a fine support for those dealing with headaches, insomnia, and a nervous stomach. To top things off, it is a great breath freshener and mouthwash if made into a tea.

The tea is made from drying the flowers and the leaves, grinding them up to the size of standard tea leaves. You then put a spoonful into a tea ball and let it soak in boiling water for about ten minutes, mixing occasionally. If you decide to take it internally, I suggest you use caution as certain medications can cause problems when combined with its use.

My wife and I also make a disinfecting spray: take 1 cup of lavender flowers, stems, and leaves mixed together. Put them in a pot with about two quarts of water. Simmer until about half of the liquid has evaporated, mixing thoroughly. Once completed, strain, let cool, and put in a spray bottle with a misting nozzle.

Now you are all set to help ward off infectious germs that might enter your home. We use it for everything from disinfecting doorknobs to cleaning air ducts. It also kills most moulds on contact and even helps in keeping mice and spiders from entering, as they don't like the scent.

If one has a stuffy nose or a cold, they can hold their head over a steaming pot of lavender and breathe deep. This helps break up congestion and supports the lungs in clearing out viruses. Laura used it daily throughout the house, as my wife does today. It's also good for cuts, scrapes, burns, insect stings, and muscle aches like rheumatism or arthritis.

To top things off, it is really easy to grow, and one can buy it in any nursery in the early spring. Two small plants will yield more than what one family could use in one year. It is one more item to put on your list when planting your gardens come spring.

Wisdom is only given to those that are willing to accept it.

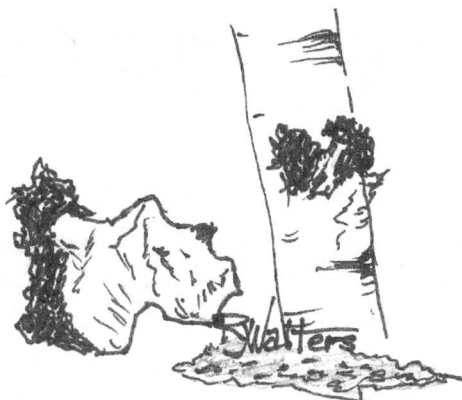

Chaga

When people get sick, they usually turn to the medical profession for prescription drugs to make them better, with very few looking at natural medicine and what it can do. One of Nature's natural medicines is Chaga. One of my sources says that Chaga is a mushroom that contains medicinal properties that some say can help strengthen and support the body naturally against many diseases.

The Chaga fungus grows on white and yellow birch trees and occasionally on hard maples. It has the highest ORAC value of any substance ever tested on the planet. (ORAC = Oxygen Radical Absorbance Capacity), measured in units of antioxidants. The ORAC value of Chaga is 35,000 compared to spinach which is 1,260 or blueberries which are 9,160. New findings now are saying that another fruit that is higher than goji berries or acai berries is, guess what? Chokecherries. Just one more super-food for us to enjoy.

Chaga tea is useful because you can apply it directly to cuts, scrapes, burns, and bruises to help the skin naturally. Only use if the Chaga has been thoroughly cleaned beforehand. I started drinking Chaga to help boost my energy levels and strengthen my immune system. In turn, I believe it helped me a lot. As I said earlier, I was diagnosed with cancer in 2010. After rigorous research, I decided to fix this problem using nothing but nature along with changing my lifestyle. The main plant that I have used in my journey is the Dandelion; that information you will find at the end of this book.

I have found drinking 1 cup of Chaga tea twice a week helps clear my mind and allows me to relax, removing anxiety almost immediately. People who have dealt with cancer should consider Chaga tea, as my sources say it can support the body in managing unhealthy cells while leaving the healthy cells unharmed. Grey Wolf's notes said for those that suffer from respiratory discomfort or asthma, a cup a day for two days would be a great asset. Other notes say that Chaga tea can also help those with fungal issues, intestinal parasites, and joint discomfort.

Reports from clinics in Vladivostok mentioned it helped with psoriasis 100%. If that is true, it would be amazing! It didn't work for me, though. Everyone is different. With all this information, it is my view that Chaga should be on the list for helping the immune system.

Precautions: There's some concern when taking Chaga in combination with blood-thinning, cholesterol, or diabetes medications, so one should check with their doctor before taking. Everyone's body works differently; try a wee bit first to see how your body reacts. And make sure your source is reliable.

Brewing Chaga tea: Simmer in chemical-free water at 100–120°F. Add 1 teaspoon of Chaga to your teapot for every 8oz of water. Let steep for 10–15 minutes. You can add a sweetener like raw coconut palm sugar or even a touch of dark cocoa. My wife and I recommend drinking Chaga only twice a month. You can reuse the grounds one more time if stored in the fridge.

Through experimentation, I found that to get the most nourishment out of Chaga, it is best to simmer it until the liquid is 25% reduced. The time to harvest is mid-winter through spring. Only take what you need, leaving the rest to flourish.

Grey Wolf said that the help in Chaga is numerous, but browsing through the bush in the middle of winter to find it gives you exercise and fresh air—which could be as good as the Chaga itself.

The secret to happiness is only a smile away.

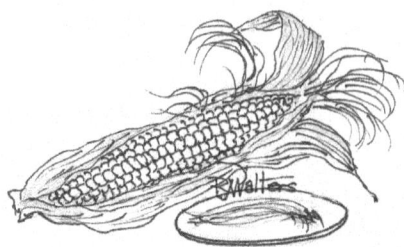

Corn Silk

Corn Silk is another part of Nature that should be in everyone's medicine chest. If for nothing else, than to have a nice hot cup of tea made from it once in a while. It has a unique flavour which keeps you wanting more. My wife and I enjoy it and make it a practice to have a cup or two at least once a month.

But let's get on to what Nature had in mind for this plant medicinally. It is best to wait until the tassel has dropped its pollen, as that way it doesn't disrupt the road that Mother Nature is following. Meaning the pollination process that will in time sprout out some of the sweetest corn this side of heaven. Or, one would hope so—barring raccoons, insects, high winds, and hail.

Once it has shed its pollen, the silk can be harvested, dried, and stored in jars for future use. Once dried, these herbs and plants can be kept for years if stored properly. Corn silk is a diuretic, which means it is a substance that promotes the production of urine. It is said that it helps with a whole range of urinary concerns.

Corn silk made into an extract is the best way to administer it. Notes say if making the extract, let it cool, then take 1/8 of a tablespoon every 3–4 hours. If made using alcohol, it will keep from spoiling for months if kept in a cool, dark place. If made from just water, store it in the fridge and use it up within a week.

You can also make a tea from the silk, which I like; you just have to make sure you get all the strands of silk removed before drinking. A filter works well. Finally, corn-silk tea is also useful for those suffering from nausea or an upset stomach.

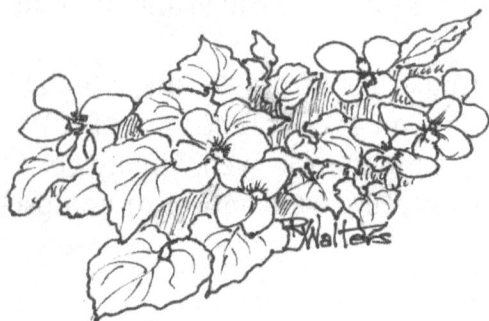

Violets

Violets are one of the most overlooked plants; most pass them by without a second glance. If you took a real close look at the leaves on the violet plant, you would soon see they resemble the human heart. That in itself should get one's attention, as it's Nature's way of letting you know that they can help you with heart-related concerns. Nature in herself is impressive. She grows where we can get at her, most of the time, along with sending out information on how she can help us without saying a word. And what happens? We just walk right on by.

Medicinal uses vary when it comes to using violets. My wife and I love to make teas using the dried leaves or petals midsummer. I also like to take the petals and mix them in with our homemade bread. They make the dough just that much better, as it helps support the body in clearing out impurities that could be in the flours of today. It also helps to keep the bread fresher, which makes a great sandwich.

Notes say a decoction made from the leaves is very good for children and adults that have problems with constipation, colds, sore throats, and flu. You can also use the roots and seeds together—dried, ground, and mixed with organic vinegar—to treat gout externally. The seeds by themselves are also very good for those suffering from stones in the kidneys and bladder. Grandad said a decoction of the entire plant could be taken for stomach pain of all kinds.

Grey Wolf said his people for many years made an infusion using the roots, soaking corn seeds just before planting, which eliminated insects that could harm the plant.

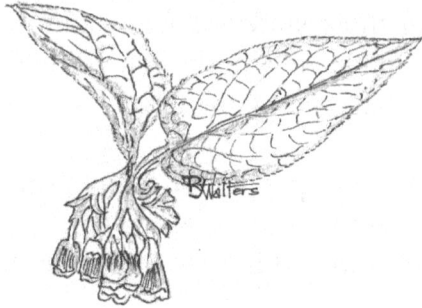

Comfrey

I love this plant, if for nothing else than its looks, and even more for what it has done to help thousands of people over the years. The Natives called it Knit-bone, as it had healed broken bones and wounds when no other medicine was able to do so. If you look at the leaf on a comfrey plant, you will see how the veins in the leaf are knitted together. Self-explanatory, really.

It grows in meadows, near springs, and in gardens. The root is the part most used and is soothing and a bit slimy. As soon as it is put on the skin, it is soaked in. Notes say that this plant is very rich in Allantoin, which helps cells grow faster. Allantoin is found in abundance in women that are pregnant, as it helps the baby grow rapidly, and it is also found in the mother's milk at first.

Once you have the roots dug, cleaned, cut, and dried, you can store them in a clean mason jar. When needed, grind up a few pieces using a mortar and pestle. You can use them alone by putting a few pieces in a glass of warm water and letting it set for a day, then rub on affected areas. Remember one thing, though: I don't recommend anyone takes comfrey internally. The Natives used it for years, but the recipes for doing this safely have been long forgotten.

Myself, I have taken it, but it consists of a meagre amount of roots ground up and made into a tea—a decoction of 1/2 to 2 ounces of the root to one quart of boiling water. The only reason I am mentioning it is so that if someone is as adventurous as myself, you will at least have a bit of information to go by with the hopes of not making yourself seriously sick.

Grey Wolf used the internal treatment for women who had severe yeast infections and for those with nasty coughs, as it promoted the discharge of mucus. (Once again, I don't recommend you use it internally.) My notes say externally it can be used once a day for no more than one week, then one should wait for two weeks before using again. The mashed roots make an excellent aid for treating bruises, ruptures, fresh wounds, skin ulcers, and gout.

It is worth mentioning that one should take great care in cleaning a wound before applying comfrey. It heals so fast it could quite possibly heal the skin right over an infection. Another way I use comfrey is to mix the roots with the leaves and a few petals. The flowers draw bees and hummingbirds to the garden for pollination.

To make a comfrey ointment: Cut your leaves, roots, and flowers into small pieces and dry them. Store in mason jars. Use one cup of dried crushed roots, one cup of dried leaves, and half a cup of dried flowers. Cover these in a jar with organic cold-pressed virgin olive oil. Put a paper towel under the outside ring to let it breathe while keeping out dust. Stir and squeeze the ingredients every couple of days. Set in a cool, dark place for two months.

You then have a great exterior treatment for backaches, psoriasis, arthritis, and muscle pains.

Nature hides her secrets so we might learn.

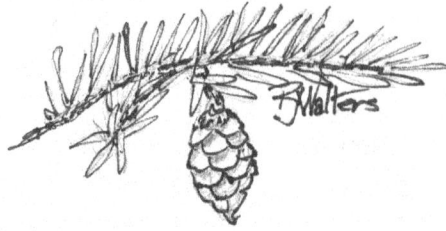

Hemlock

This tree for years has helped many with all kinds of problems. It can reach a height of 80 feet if left undisturbed. Grey Wolf's notes say a decoction of the bark can be made, which is an excellent wash for a condition traditionally called falling of the womb.

Oil of hemlock years ago was used externally for treating rheumatism, sciatica, and for lumbago. My findings are that it should be used externally only and never used internally. On the subject of lumbago: it seems nowadays that the medical profession doesn't even acknowledge lumbago. Years ago it was known by many and easily treated, as one knew what it was that was bothering them.

Today folks have been told they have numerous problems when in reality it is just one problem: lumbago. An explanation of lumbago years ago would consist of this: My friend, you have a backache affecting the lumbar region or lower back. This can be caused by muscle strain or arthritis or vascular insufficiency—which means the blood is blocked in the area that is hurting, not being able to flow freely—or a ruptured part of a disc. Most of which is caused by hard work over the years and aging.

The treatment for this as stated in Grey Wolf's notes is as follows: Take 3 ounces of hemlock bark to 1 quart of boiling water. You can boil it for an hour, or you can boil it for a half hour, depending on what strength you wish to make. I like mine stronger in the beginning, then easing off to a mild solution once the problem is on the mend. Remember: never take this internally. Now apply the wash to the area in need three to four times a day until better.

Seems to me, it would be worth a try. Your choice though.

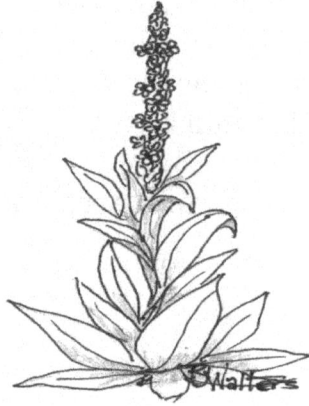

Mullen

Natives and naturalists have used this plant for years.
There isn't much it doesn't do. My notes are as follows. For
those that have chronic ear pain, come summer when the
Mullein plant comes out into bloom, head on out and gather up
a bunch of petals and let them dry.

You then take enough petals to fill a small mason jar. You
can also add one small clove of dried garlic to the mixture, as
this will aid in its effectiveness. Then fill the jar with extra
virgin, cold-pressed olive oil. Cover the jar and place in the
sunlight for three days. Stir occasionally using a wooden spoon
to release the air bubbles. Once ready, strain well and put into
smaller jars, adding two drops of vitamin E to each jar and
seal. Store in a cool, dry place or the fridge. It will last for
about one month.

When needed, use a dropper to put two drops into the ear
that hurts. Lay on your side and let the drops run in, then put a
clean cotton ball just inside to keep the oil from leaking out. It
is also great for earwax buildup; two drops in each ear twice a
day for two days usually corrects the problem. Ladies can also
use it to treat irritated or infected ear piercings.

A tea is made by simmering 4 ounces of fresh or 6 ounces of dry leaves in one pint of milk for 10 minutes. This is very good for helping those with external discomforts like hemorrhoids; use it as a wash, straining well before using. It is also said that a poultice made from the pulp and leaves works well for treating sprains and swellings.

You can also make a weak tea using the mullein leaves, which is good for those with weak eyes or cataracts. Use one spoonful of crushed dried leaves per cup of hot water. You must strain this very well using an unbleached organic coffee filter to remove every tiny hair, then cool and rinse the eyes twice a day. The leaves infused in hot water and vinegar are also very good for gargling to help with sore throats and tonsillitis. Discard the liquid after gargling and do not use the vinegar solution in your eyes.

Mullein roots and leaves were traditionally smoked to help with lung congestion and asthma. One must first dry the leaves or roots and grind them to a coarse blend. Care should be taken, though, as Grey Wolf said the veins in the leaves, when smoked, can have a light-headed or hallucinating effect for some. My grandfather said for those that want to stop smoking tobacco, this would be of great help as it calms the mind.

You can also use the soft leaves in your shoes or boots to soothe aching feet or to help with athlete's foot. Some have even used the leaves as a substitute for toilet paper, but I don't recommend it. There are tiny hairs on the leaves which, for some, cause a terrible rash.

Fantasies are unborn realities.

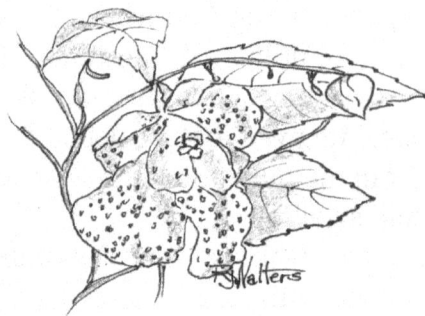

Jewel Weed

Jewel weed is a plant that, if found and identified, would save days if not weeks of grief, as it is a natural antidote for those suffering from poison ivy. It is also very good for stopping the itch caused by stinging nettles, poison oak, insect bites, burns, cuts, eczema, and acne.

There isn't much preparation needed for treating these conditions other than finding the plant, breaking a piece of the stem, and putting the juice on the affected area. This is one of the best remedies for poison ivy known to man. It grows almost everywhere in Ontario and most of the USA, usually in moist areas in the shade. The flowers are orange-red with red spots and are trumpet-shaped, blooming from early summer to fall. They are a touch under one inch long with three petals, one of which curls to form a long, slipper-shaped spur.

The leaves have a waxy surface coating that repels water, and the veins in the leaves stop at the notches. Stems are semitransparent, meaning you can see the light through them. The bottoms of the leaves when underwater take on a silvery colour—it looks pretty, and once you see it, you will never forget it.

Ripe jewel weed seed pods are exceptionally delicate. The slightest touch causes them to burst, scattering their seeds over a large area. Each seed inside the pods is about the size of unground pepper.

If you can catch some seeds, it would be in your best interest to take some home and plant them nearby for those emergencies that will inevitably come your way. To catch them, wrap your hand around the pods, leaving no room for the seeds to escape when they explode. Some ingredients in jewel weed are similar to those found in commercial treatments for inflammation, but without the added chemicals. It is loaded with anti-inflammatory and antihistamine properties, which is why it works so efficiently on skin problems.

As I stated, it grows mostly in wet, shady areas, but if one finds poison ivy, chances are jewel weed will be growing nearby. It seems Mother Nature has plants that can cause problems, but she also readily gives you the cure if you take the time to seek out what she has to offer. How jewel weed got its name is that when water lies on the top of the leaves, they look like shimmering jewels. It is a great piece of Nature that everyone should have in their medicine chest or at the very least know where it grows.

There is more to Nature than we are being told or led to believe.

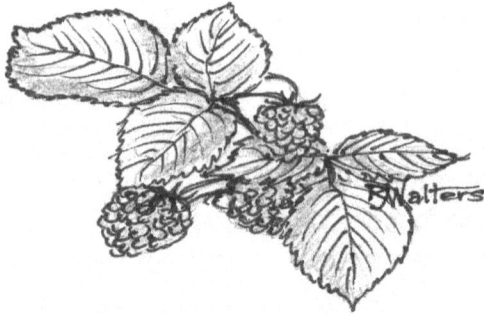

Raspberry Leaves

There are all kinds of raspberries throughout the world, and most have the same properties. The fruit they produce by itself is healthy for the body. Raspberries are very rich in Vitamin C; just one small cup provides up to about 90% of the daily needs to keep us healthy. It is a great detoxifier, helping the body clear out impurities in large quantities when eaten fresh.

My Grandmother helped many a woman that was in the family-way, giving them raspberry tea made with the leaves, as it strengthens and helps to tone the uterine tissue. This assists contractions and keeps in check any bleeding during labour. Around four cups a day when in labour would be appropriate. You can make an infusion using 1 ounce of the dried leaves in a pint of water; bring to a boil and then simmer for ten to fifteen minutes.

Grey Wolf also used the tea to support the body during asthma, colds, coughs, and digestive issues like diarrhea. He also said one could smoke it in a pipe or burn it in a smudge pot, meaning that when inhaled, it had a spiritual or mystic power for many and was used when tobacco was unavailable. The leaves were also dried and placed on sweat stones in saunas, which helped with sore throats, chills, and detoxing of the skin.

I, for one, have used the leaves made into a tea for treating cataracts. I treated myself with excellent results, and others I have known have had excellent results as well. The treatment consists of around three or four leaves, dried or fresh, along with a spoonful of rose petals. Wild roses are excellent; don't use the ones you buy in a store as they have been sprayed with chemicals.

Boil some water, pour it into a cup, and add the leaves and petals. Let sit for about ten minutes. Once cool, strain thoroughly and rinse eyes with the solution two times a day for one week—once in the morning and once before bedtime. One thing to take into account: never use the same solution for both eyes, as it could spread the condition you are trying to fix. Also, when straining, use an organic coffee filter for best results. Not the white coloured ones, as they have been bleached.

I have found that for some, the first time it burns a touch, but with each treatment, the feeling is less. I would suggest you make a very weak solution to start off with and ease into it. Also, as with any plants, try a bit of the solution on your wrist first. If it turns red or itchy, then you are allergic to it and shouldn't use it. In saying that, I haven't found any plants to date that I am allergic to—even poison ivy doesn't affect me. Everyone is different, though. Last but not least, raspberries are very alkaline, which is great for raising the pH in the body.

Nature is our true direction. To fear it, we cloud the way.

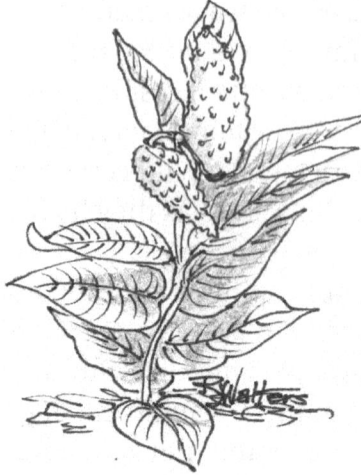

Milk Weed

Here again is a plant that most just take for granted. It grows in specific areas throughout North America, making itself readily available to all those that choose to use its incredible powers. To start off, my notes say it can be used to increase the secretion of bile from the liver and gallbladder. It is also useful for gallstones, stomach, and urinary concerns.

If one made a decoction from the roots, it would help immensely with those suffering from dropsy—an old-fashioned term for swelling caused by fluid buildup. I remember one time Grey Wolf fixing up a solution for a fellow that lived up the road from us; he was suffering from rheumatism so badly he could hardly get out of bed. After fixing up what he called the cure, within one week the old feller was dancing up a storm.

The decoction consists of 4–8 ounces of dried roots boiled in 6 quarts of rainwater. He insisted it had to be rainwater, saying the ingredients in it make the roots twice as potent (just make sure your rainwater is clean and fresh). Once made, you take

2–4 ounces three times a day until you feel better. Store the remainder in the fridge and discard after four days.

Others say that if you were to squish a leaf and piece of stem, the juices help with sores and skin bruises, like psoriasis. The milk that comes from the stem is excellent for warts and moles. Grey Wolf treated many people using the milky sap of milkweed for swollen joints and arthritic ailments.

He also would take the white part of the plant and mix it with a little water so it would go down easier—about a spoonful to a half-cup of water once a day, taken for four days. He says it helps those with hip problems, swollen knees, and degenerated discs. One must be careful with the milk, however, as it can be very irritating if it gets into the eyes.

Using Nature opens the doors to reality.

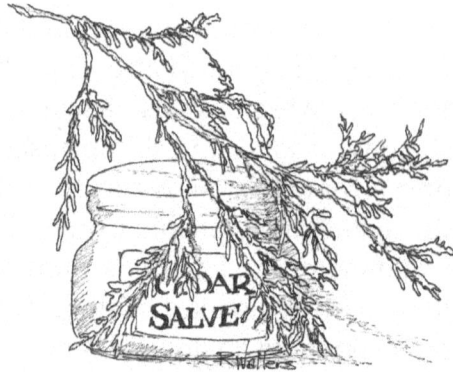

Cedar

Cedar is a tree that most think is only used for its wood to build things. I have used white cedar for a number of items, including my Native American Flutes, as there is no better wood for making them.

But let's talk medicinal uses. First, I believe that before one uses the natural medicines of today, one should clear their minds of all negative thinking, which is where cedar comes into play. Over the years I have tried to stay within grasping distance of the culture and beliefs of years ago. Whether it be foraging, hunting, or farming, I know how powerful the clearing of one's mind can be.

What I like to do is gather some cedar bark or leaves and dry them. I then put a cup full into a steel container, add a couple of tablespoons of sage, and light it. The smoke itself will help clear one's mind of ill thoughts and replenishes what is needed to help solve the problems at hand. This is also a good time to ask the smoke for help in other areas of despair.

Then sit back and feel what takes place in your mind and soul. Cedar and sage smoke has been used for centuries by our ancestors, and I continue to use it myself. Be prepared, as the smoke reveals everything and allows nothing to be hidden for those that choose to believe in it.

Now that the mind has been taken care of, you can use the cedar for getting well. My favourite is the treatment for arthritis or rheumatism. The tincture consists of two cups of dried cedar leaves, one spoonful of lavender, and one teaspoonful of sage. Put these in a small jar and cover with one part organic cold-pressed olive oil to one part vodka. Use only vodka that comes in a glass bottle, never from a plastic container.

Cover the leaves with the solution, put a lid on (not too tight), and store in a cool, dark place for three months. Mark the date on the bottle so you don't forget. Cedar is also used for eliminating moths and spiders from your home. Laura years ago always hung a few pieces in her closets, which saved many a good dress from moths—not to forget the surprise of a hairy spider in your sweater.

It is also excellent used externally for the discomfort of inflammation in the hands, back, legs, or neck, as it is a potent anti-inflammatory. It is also a very good antiseptic and works well in treating cold sores. These remedies are for external use only. Don't forget to thank Nature when gathering her treasures and never take more than you need.

One learns through the ear, not the tongue.

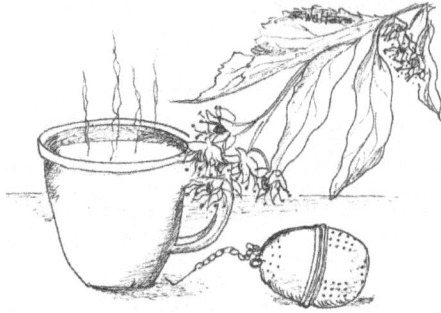

Basswood Tree

Basswood or as some call it the Linden Tree. This tree is amongst the greatest of healers. It can live up to 200 years old. Imagine the stories they could tell us. The wood in itself is white and soft. If put on water, it would float like a cork. They grow in abundance throughout North America, being more pronounced around the Great Lakes.

When in bloom, the scent they give off cannot be missed as it carries on the breezes for miles, which not only tells us where they are living but also the birds, animals, and bees. It is a smell like no other, enticing one to stop and take in its aroma, then savouring it like a fine cup of perked organic coffee. For years my German friends and family have used different parts of the tree to treat many ailments. Poultices can be made from the large leaves and bark.

There is another set of leaves—**long, narrow, and pointed —that sprouts out with blossoms hanging from their centre.** I was told these two narrow leaves were used to treat a fever. They also have the potential to clear our sinuses.

My wife and I have used the basswood blossoms for many years treating our colds and flu with great success. A couple of blooms along with one leaf made into a tea would go a long way in the prevention of all colds and flu.

The easiest way to make a tea from the leaves or flowers is to buy yourself a tea ball. Ours is stainless steel and it unscrews from the centre. We put in what it holds in one half, mostly blossoms and one leaf. Put it back together and let it soak in a cup of boiling water for around ten minutes, moving it around occasionally.

Three cups a day for three days at the first signs of a cold or flu taking place.

If the blossoms are left on the tree, they will turn into hard nut-like seeds. If these are allowed to mature they can be taken into the house, dried, crushed, and used to make a chocolatey tasting drink. It is very delicious.

Problems arise, though, as the birds, chipmunks, and squirrels also know how good these are, and one has to be quick in getting to them before they do.

To heal ones-self one must first find the strengths from within.

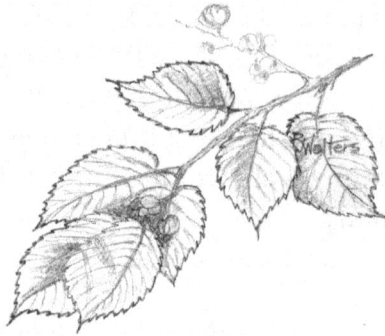

Slippery Elm

Grey Wolf made an oil mixed with the slippery elm's inner bark together with the inner bark of the willow tree. Pussy-willows were okay to use if regular willows weren't available. He used this for treating all kinds of muscle pain, torn ligaments, arthritis, rheumatism, lower back pain, prostate pain, sore arms and legs, neck pains, tendinitis, along with helping immensely for those suffering with hemorrhoids or piles.

Here is what is stated in his notes: Take one handful of slippery elm inner bark dried, cut up into small pieces; 1/2 cup of the inner bark from the willow; 4 tbs of lavender (either stems, flowers or leaves); 4 tbs of Calendula petals; and 4 tbs of either violet petals, leaves or a mix of each. Now you take all your ingredients, put them in your jar, mix together and cover with oil. Fill the jar and let it set in a cool dark place for one month before using. Stir occasionally. He didn't mention the kind of oil; if it was me making it, I would use a good brand of extra virgin, cold-pressed olive oil.

For the cap, use the outer ring putting a piece of cloth over the mason jar. This allows things to breathe. Never seal it completely. This is only for external treatments; do not take it internally. Now, a bit on the inner bark of the slippery elm: it is called cambium, which is a thin layer of tissue lying between the bark and the wood of a stem.

In the spring, when the tree is just starting to show itself, the cambium is the thickest and this is when it should be harvested. Remember though, Nature is there for all to enjoy, and to take everything and leave nothing isn't the right thing to do. Take what you need and always leave more than you take, so that Nature can carry on and flourish.

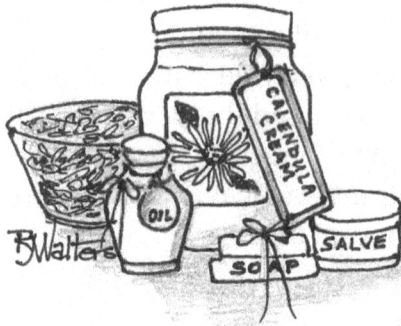

Calendula

Calendula has been used for a good number of years for different ailments along with making a great-tasting tea. It is easy to grow and, once planted, will return every year. My wife and I have used them in treating all kinds of different ailments. Not many folks know this, but they really help those with varicose veins. The Calendula helps to strengthen the capillary and vein walls which are weak in varicose veins. Its anti-inflammatory properties are also useful here.

Grey Wolf used yarrow, lavender, and witch hazel along with Calendula in a mixture to treat varicose veins along with a great number of other problems. The yarrow helps to promote the circulation of blood, helping the body clear any old blood in the veins. The lavender oil adds healing and anti-inflammatory properties that can help with the itching that is associated with varicose veins.

The witch hazel has been used for varicose veins for years as it tends to shrink or constrict body tissues, which is what is needed. Witch hazel grows in the eastern part of the country from Ontario to Nova Scotia. It can also be found in a lot of health food stores.

Grey Wolf said the best way to make the tincture is to fill a mason jar with half-dried Calendula flowers and half-dried yarrow. If yarrow is not available, fill the jar with the dried Calendula flowers on their own, or if you have dried violet flowers, use them in place of the yarrow.

Now if available put in some witch hazel—a handful is sufficient—and cover with a good vodka and let set for three weeks, shaking or stirring with a wooden spoon daily. After three weeks you should strain and add 10–30 drops of lavender essential oil per quart of spray. Pour the solution into a spray bottle and label it with the date. This now can be sprayed on varicose veins as often as desired. For your face, spray some on your hands (clean of course) and gently massage into the problem area.

If directions are followed correctly, you should see some good results. Don't forget, as with any natural potions, rub a wee bit on your wrist and see if it turns red or gets itchy. If so, as I have stated many times, you are allergic to it and care should be taken. I say care, as sometimes the body has to adjust to the tincture and can still be used a little at a time until it becomes accustomed to its effects. If it gets too red and itchy, discontinue use.

My Grandfather used to say the world is getting jammed up like pickles in a barrel.

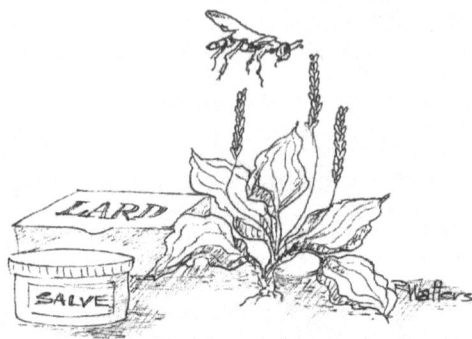

Plantain

Through my research over the years, I have learned that plantain can help with many health-related concerns, such as urinary infections, ulcers, or other gastrointestinal inflammations. For making medicines, I recommend harvesting the whole plant, including the roots, flower, stalk, and seeds. Dry them naturally and put them in jars for future use.

What is impressive is its ability to draw out poisons and infections from wounds. It can be used in severe cases such as a rattlesnake bite or blood poisoning (while also seeking medical help, of course). It can also be used for bee stings and spider bites. I like to use it as a tea, tincture, oil, or salve. If in season, the fresh plantain "spit poultice" works best.

The spit poultice consists of clean, raw plantain from a chemical-free area. Place the leaf into your mouth and chew it slightly so that it releases its juices. Chew it into a ball and then spit it onto a clean hand. Now place the poultice on the affected area. If possible, I add a fresh one about every fifteen minutes; if it starts to feel warm on the wound, that is a signal that it's time to apply a new batch.

Here in parts of North America in the spring, black flies invade us. These pesky critters not only bite, but they take a whole piece along with them. Then comes the itch, which in some cases can last for weeks. The worst thing one can do is scratch it. I have seen young ones scratch until the bite starts to bleed. If a person would immediately chew up a piece of plantain and apply it to the bite, the itch would leave quite quickly and save a lot of grief.

It also works well on mosquito bites, stopping the itch within a minute or two. My notes say that plantain also helps those that have problems urinating, as it promotes the body to produce and eliminate water naturally. My Grandfather used it for hemorrhoids with irritation. To identify plantain, find someone who knows the plant or check a reliable source.

Once determined, you will have no problem finding them in your lawn or garden. Just make sure it is a clean, chemical-free area. My Dad used to say that we are people who thrive on explanations.

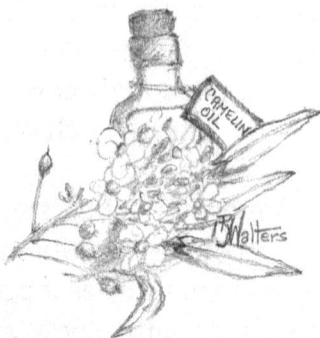

Camelina

Here is one plant that I believe is going to bring us some fantastic healing properties in the near future. Research is only beginning to realize just how vital it can be. LC-PUFA (long-chain polyunsaturated fatty acids) consists of omega-3, omega-6, and many other properties, some just starting to show themselves.

The best part is that this substance can be gotten from the plant called Camelina. I have long believed that most of the people today are lacking significantly in omega-3 and omega-6. With our bodies lacking these, I think we've invited in a whole mess of diseases and health-related issues. Grey Wolf many years ago used this plant, saying all that is needed is the want to go out and gather it. He suggested adding the seeds of the plant to the food we eat.

Today it is being made into an oil. It is quite expensive and not readily found in grocery stores, but it is out there if you choose to seek it out. I believe that it should be incorporated back into our lifestyle. The other thing I like about it is that the omega-3 and 6 it contains arrives from a plant and not from fish.

Putting things together, I would say it would be a great support for those that have leukemia, prostate, or breast concerns, along with helping the body manage infections, arthritis, diabetes, osteoporosis, and inflammatory ailments. Two other benefits would be the healthy development of the brain along with improving our eyesight.

When buying, make sure it hasn't been altered through GMO. This is very important. Raw organic, cold-pressed would be my choice.

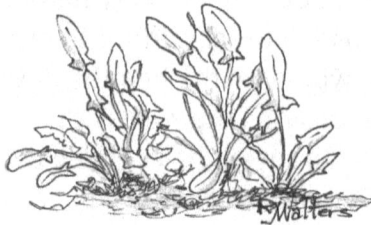

Sheep Sorrel

Sheep sorrel I have found can help those with sore throats if made into a tea and used to gargle with. It is also useful for internal and external bleeding due to its sour, bitter taste.

It is very high in antioxidants which protect the cells in our body from free-radical damage caused by pollutants and the general destruction of our cells which occurs daily. Research says it is a very good antiseptic, antibacterial, antiviral, and anti-parasitic. It also seems to be helpful for those with tumours, which would be a great support for those dealing with cancer.

It also has quite high anti-inflammatory properties, which in my mind would make it a real asset for those who have arthritis. Sheep sorrel in most areas is also high in selenium which comes from the soil it grows in (different soil, of course, would reflect on how much selenium was in the plant). Knowing that selenium is very good for those who have cancer and other diseases, I would then think that sheep sorrel would be great to add to a salad now and then. Selenium is also high in tomatoes.

You can always identify sheep sorrel by its distinct arrow-shaped leaves if you are unsure, or you can look it up on the internet. The sour taste helps with its identification. I like to eat it raw whenever I come upon it.

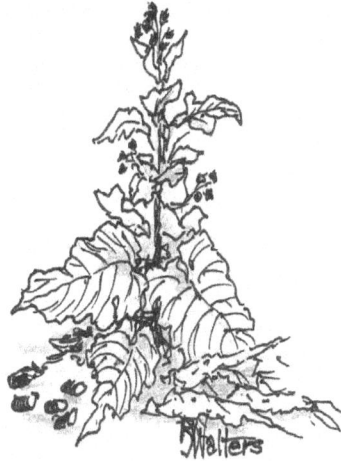

Burdock Root

Burdock grows pretty well everywhere, and it isn't hard to find. The parts I use mostly are the roots. When digging the roots, they should be cut into tiny pieces and dried. It is essential to cut them before they are dried, as once dried it is almost impossible to grind or cut. I found that out from experience.

The burdock is easily identified with its large rhubarb-like leaves, along with having burs that stick tight to one's clothing. This is the way it transports itself to other areas. Pretty ingenious on its part. It does have a lot of medicinal properties. It promotes sweating and urination and is very cleansing. It is also used for blood-related concerns. It is also excellent as a support in the treatment of various types of cancer.

Grey Wolf's notes said that the seeds, when taken and pounded into a powder, also help to increase the flow of urine. The dosage one should consider is 1/2 to 1 teaspoonful twice a day. A decoction or tea is supposed to be very good for rheumatism, gout, and other blood-related issues. I have found, though, it works a lot better if you mix it with dandelion roots.

The decoction is made by boiling 4 ounces of the root, adding an ounce of dandelion roots to one quart of water. The seeds promote urine more so than the roots and are a better alternative in treating kidney troubles. Grey Wolf made a poultice from the leaves and applied it to skin sores and leg ulcers with great success. I have found the same application can be used for treating acne. The older leaves are the ones to use, as they hold more healthy properties than the younger leaves.

He also said a tea made from the roots is excellent for gallbladder problems and it is very healing for the liver. The root tea also can help the body eliminate gallstones and kidney stones, he says. Burdock root tea tastes like its name: rooty.

The cure for any disease starts at the root.

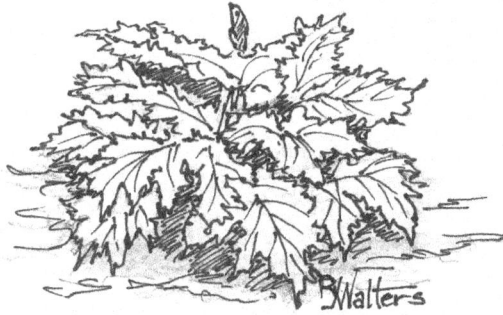

Turkey Rhubarb

Turkey rhubarb, or as some would call it, Indian rhubarb or wild rhubarb. Rhubarb is about the most interesting part of the Essiac recipe. Most don't understand the concept behind what went into the tea. Myself, I believe—though not proven, of course—that Rene Caisse, in the beginning, used regular rhubarb roots along with wild rhubarb which at the time was plentiful for her mixture in treating cancer. Later on, it was possible for her to obtain turkey rhubarb from different countries; whether she did or not, no one will ever really know.

In my thinking and usage, I have found that rhubarb, be it roots or stalk, has a laxative effect on one's body. I believe that Grey Wolf dried the roots of the rhubarb adding it to his treatments, if for nothing else than to keep the body eliminating toxins. If you look at some of his recipes, you will notice that he uses only one ounce at a time, which is next to nil, but still enough to keep one regular, which would have been an essential part in getting well.

Remember never eat the leaves, as they are quite poisonous on the rhubarb plant. In saying that, a person would have to ingest quite a few leaves for it to be fatal, but just the same, leave them alone. If you are in need of a laxative, I would suggest you just eat a couple of bowls of rhubarb stalks—boiled and cooled in the fridge mixed with a touch of sweetener like organic coconut palm sugar.

It is said that you can dye your hair using rhubarb roots. For many years, Native women used the roots of the rhubarb to lighten their hair. The recipe for that consists of two cups of roots, simmered with just enough water to cover them for one-half hour. Then add a bit of the leaves, which will darken the mixture to your liking. Now let it set overnight.

Remember though: if you do put it on your hair, it is permanent, so care should be taken. You can also use the mixture to dye your wool or clothes. Experiment and you will come up with all kinds of colours and, best of all, it is all natural.

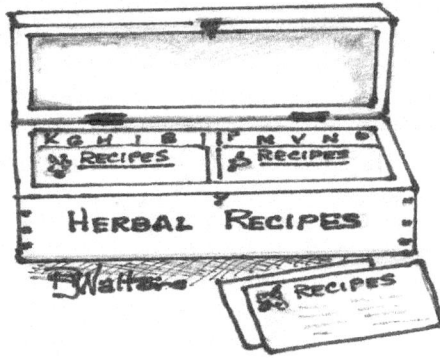

Herbal Recipes

Grey Wolf's Notes

Over the years, Grey Wolf has used a significant number of different items consisting of plants and trees with healing properties. Listed below are a few of his favourites. For information on how to make decoctions and infusions, refer to the section: How herbs and plants are made into medicine. Gallstones: Decoctions & Infusions

The Northern Forest Blend

3 tsp Milk Thistle Seeds (crushed)

2 tsp Stinging Nettle Leaf

2 tsp Dandelion Leaf

1 tsp Dandelion Root

1 tsp Birch Leaf

— This makes 1 quart.

— Take internally, 1 cup per day for two weeks, sipping throughout the day.

— Note on Safety: This blend is designed to get bile moving. If you have a large stone or a blocked duct, do not use these herbs. Forcing the gallbladder to contract against a blockage can cause a medical emergency. Use this for maintenance only; if in active pain, see a doctor.

Burdock Root for Gallstones

Grey Wolf gave chopped burdock root to those with gallstones who were unable to eat because food made them sick.
— Use the roots to make a tea.
— Place a few cut pieces in boiling water and steep for 10 minutes.
— Results are typically seen within a few days.

Liver Complaints: Decoctions & Infusions

2 tsp Milk Thistle Seeds (crushed)
2 tsp Dandelion Root
1 tsp Peppermint Leaf
1/2 tsp Caraway Seed (crushed)
— Make 1 quart.
— Take 2 cups per day for two weeks, sipping throughout the day.

Nasal Rinse

1/4 tsp Iodized Salt
8 oz Glass of Water
— Mix thoroughly.
— Use in the morning and before going to bed.

Healing Salve (For All Sores)

1 tsp Calendula blossoms
2 tsp Plantain leaf
2 tsp Comfrey leaf
— Mix into a base for an amazing healing salve.

Chest Infection & Cough Syrup

This recipe encourages a healthy fever and helps the body deal with common bacteria and viruses. It makes an excellent cough syrup.

1 full Garlic bulb, regular size
4 inch piece of Ginger root
2 tbs Fennel seeds
1 cup Apple Cider Vinegar
1/2 cup Local Honey
— Store in the fridge once made; good for one week.
— Dose is 1 teaspoon, 1 to 3 times a day or as needed.

Dandelion Soup

4 potatoes, peeled and sliced
6 cups water
1 tbs Sea Salt (or less, to taste)
1/2 pound Dandelion leaves and stems, rinsed
2 egg yolks
1 tbs Butter (the best you can find)
— Place the sliced potatoes in the water.
— Add salt and cook 15 minutes over medium heat.
— Add the dandelion leaves and simmer 15 minutes more.
— Beat together the egg yolks and butter, then stir into the soup for 1 minute.
— Serve hot with homemade bread.
— Pick dandelions as early as possible in the spring for tenderness.

Dandelion Root Broth

Grey Wolf made a broth of dandelion roots, stewing them in hot water with sorrel and the yolk of an egg.

— Taken daily for a month, this helped those with diabetes.

— This broth also helps with liver problems, kidneys, and the urinary tract.

Gooseberry Pudding

Great for diabetes and inflammation of the pancreas.

3 tbs Cornstarch

1 cup Water

1 quart Gooseberries

2 cups Raw Organic Coconut Palm Sugar

— Dissolve cornstarch in the water in a saucepan.

— Add gooseberries and sugar; cook until thickened.

— Serve warm as a tasty treat.

Chokecherry Sauce

Warning: Never consume the seeds of the chokecherry as they contain cyanide and are poisonous. Pits must be removed completely.

1 quart Chokecherries

4 tbs Sugar (or Coconut Palm Sugar)

1 tsp Almond extract (or Vanilla)

— Wash and drain the cherries.

— Mash them whole in a strong bowl and remove every pit.

— Pour the pulp through a sieve into a saucepan.

— Add sugar and extract; simmer for 15 minutes.

Sweet Rose Hip Sauce

Rose hips are a natural source of Vitamin C and have been used for stomach disorders, circulation, and immune support.

2 cups Rose Hips, seeded

2 cups Water

1/4 cup Organic Honey

1/2 cup Turnip Flour (or 2 tbs Cornstarch)
— Cook rose hips in water until soft (about 20 minutes).
— Add honey and flour.
— Cook on low heat for another 20 minutes, stirring constantly.
— You can make turnip flour by drying and grinding turnips in a coffee grinder.

Rose Hip Sauce for Meat

Excellent with roasted venison or beef.
2 cups Rose Hips, seeded
1 1/2 cups Water
1/2 cup Raw Organic Coconut Palm Sugar
3 tbs Cornstarch
1/2 cup White Wine (optional)
— Simmer rose hips in water for 1 hour.
— Add sugar and cook for 5 more minutes.
— Add cornstarch and simmer for 3 minutes, stirring constantly.
— Add wine just before serving.

Mint Tea (Wild or Home-grown)

Used for colds, digestion, and gas.
1 quart Water
1 cup Mint leaves and blossoms
Honey or Coconut Palm Sugar (optional)
— Boil water and add mint.
— Let sit for 10 minutes.
— Sweeten to taste.
— Can also be used cold as a poultice for skin rashes.

Sage for Bleeding and Infection

Sage can stop bleeding quickly, but it should be used with caution internally as it can strain the liver in high amounts.

— To stop bleeding or treat infection externally: Boil sage in water for 15 minutes, cool, and apply the liquid to the wound.

— Internal use: Limit to one half-cup of sage tea per day, for a maximum of two days.

Homemade Apple Cider Vinegar

Apple peelings or cores
  1 tbs Sugar per cup of water
  Water
  Glass quart jar
— Fill the jar 3/4 full with apple scraps.

— Dissolve sugar in water and pour over apples, leaving a few inches of room at the top.

— Cover loosely with a paper towel and set in a warm, dark place for two weeks.

— Stir occasionally and skim off any scum.

— Strain after two weeks, then let the liquid set for another 2–4 weeks until the taste is right.

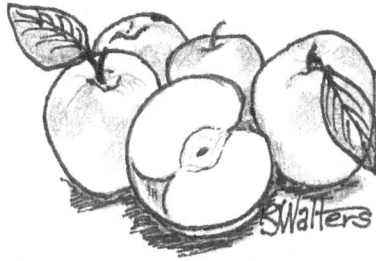

Simplified Treatments

Remember, never use pesticides or chemicals on soil or plants you plan to eat. Never harvest plants by the roadside and always identify the plant with certainty before using.

Aches & Pains
Slippery elm mixed with comfrey root was made into a tincture and used externally.
— Warning: Comfrey is for external use only. Never take internally as it can cause severe liver damage.

Acne
Avoid sugar, coffee, tea, alcohol, and junk food. Drinking dandelion tea once a week is helpful.
— To prepare: Dig up one dandelion, roots and all. Wash, grind, and put in a tea ball.
— Soak in boiling water for five minutes.
— Topical Iodine: A single drop of antiseptic iodine on a pimple can eliminate it overnight, though it stings.

Abscess
Burdock: Roots and leaves used internally and externally. (Avoid if pregnant or nursing).
Echinacea: Roots chewed, used in tea, or pulverized for external use.

Chamomile: Used in teas for sleep or applied as a wash to affected areas.

White Pine: Inner bark and young shoots used as an infusion externally. Not recommended for internal use.
Slippery Elm: Inner bark used as an infusion or tincture applied externally.

ADHD (Behavioural Support)
Treatment should entail counselling and close parental supervision.
— Lavender: Has potential for calming. Used as a mist throughout the house.
— Note: When using essential oils as a mist, ensure the area is well-ventilated and safe for children.

Headache & Allergies
Mint: Dried leaves in tea or fresh leaves in food.
Rooibos: Used as a tea.

Alzheimer's Support
Cold-pressed organic coconut oil has been used with success as both food and medicine.

Natural Antibiotics & Antiseptics
Antibiotics: Olive leaf, papaya, thyme, and raw garlic.
Antiseptics: Grapefruit (seeds, pulp, inner rind), Mint (leaves and stems), and Lavender.
Staghorn Sumac: Flower boiled for tea or made into a tincture.

White Willow: Inner bark or leaves made into a tea. Use sparingly (no more than half a cup a day).

Anxiety
Lavender: Use as a mist throughout the home to calm the environment.

Aphrodisiacs

Lavender: Mist on pillows before retiring.
Coffee: Can have a significant effect on the mind; organic decaf often works as well as caffeinated.
Marijuana: Used for years by those who know its benefits.
Savory: A fragrant herb used with excellent results.

Appetite Stimulants
Dandelion: One small plant (flower, stem, leaves, and roots) washed, chopped, and made into tea once a day.
Fennel: Seeds, leaves, and roots used in cooking or tea.
Ginger Root: Fresh pieces steeped in hot water for fifteen minutes.
Lemon Balm: Used as a calming hot tea.
Sage: Used in cooking or as a tea for digestive help.
Wild Black Cherry: Dried inner bark used in teas or syrups.

Arthritis
Ginger Root: Fresh, dried, or ground and added to food or tea.
Montmorency Sour Cherries: Eating a handful a day or drinking sugar-free juice. These naturally reduce inflammation.
Slippery Elm: Inner bark made into a tincture or oil for external use.
Garlic: One clove raw or three cooked daily, unless it causes nausea.

Asthma
Hemp: Roots boiled into teas for medicinal use.
Mullein: The oldest herb for this. Use as a tea (one cup a day). While traditionally smoked, tea is the safer recommendation.
Staghorn Sumac: Flower made into tea or oil and applied to the chest.
Black Cherry Bark: Dried inner bark used in tea or syrups.

Colds & Flu
Basswood Blossoms: The best for halting a cold. Use one spoonful of blossoms and one leaf for a cup of tea.
— Warning: Check with a doctor if you are on other medications before using Basswood.
Ginger Root: Used as a seasoning or tea to ward off or treat illness.
Onion: Eaten raw or cooked. Inhaling freshly cut onions is also a traditional aid.

Gum, Lip & Mouth Problems
Raspberry: Leaves and fruit made into a tea and used as a mouthwash.
Staghorn Sumac: Dried flower tea used as a rinse or gargle twice a day.
Willow: Bark or leaf tea used as a wash for infected areas.
Dry Lips: A traditional fix is using the natural oils from behind the ears.

Earaches
Mullein: 2–5 drops of mullein oil or tincture to soften wax or treat infection.
Onion: For swimmer's ear, a steamed, softened onion half held over the ear (once cooled enough to touch).

Urinary Tract Infections (UTI)

Prevention: Drink 8 cups of water daily and urinate regularly. Avoid sugar, alcohol, and caffeine during infection.

Treatment: Raw organic cranberries, crushed and boiled into a drink. Two cups a day and one before bed.

— Parsley and Corn Silk tea (limit to two cups a day) are also beneficial.

Yeast Infections

Treatment: Tea of mullein leaf, raspberry leaf, or garden sage. The Best: Crushed organic raw cranberries, boiled and drank once cool.

— Probiotics (Acidophilus) are highly recommended.

— Suppository: 3–5 drops of lavender essential oil on a tampon.

Lowering Blood Pressure

Garlic: One raw clove or two cooked cloves daily.

Ginger Root: Made into a tea before bedtime.

— Warning: If on pharmaceutical heart or blood pressure medication, consult a doctor before using ginger or garlic medicinally.

Honey & Cinnamon: One cup of organic honey and cinnamon water in the morning.

Circulatory Health

Burdock: Roots dried and ground; one spoonful per two cups of tea. (Avoid if pregnant).

Ginseng: Use for no more than 3 months (Asian) or 2 months (Siberian) at a time. Steep 3–5 slices for 5 minutes.

Rosemary: Use in low doses.

— Warning: High doses of rosemary can cause spasms or fluid in the lungs and can trigger miscarriages. Avoid if pregnant.

Wild Black Cherry: Dried inner bark made into tea or syrup.

Eczema & Psoriasis

Comfrey Root: Soak root in warm water overnight and apply to clean skin.

— Warning: External use only.

Elder: Ointments made from leaves or roots for bruises and irritations.

Marshmallow Root: Infusion or oil applied externally.

Sweet Potato: Eaten cooked to help from the inside.

Gallbladder & Gout

Dandelion: Eaten raw or as a tea.

Radishes: Eaten raw daily to help remove stones.

Montmorency Sour Cherries: A handful a day helps immensely with gout by reducing uric acid.

Kidney Stones & Health

Dandelion: Whole plant tea.

Wild Carrot: Dried or fresh tea, two cups a day.

Sunlight: Grey Wolf noted that Vitamin D from sunshine is essential for calcium absorption; without it, calcium accumulates into stones and plaque.

Rheumatism

Burdock: Root tea, one cup a day after eating.

Comfrey: Root soaked overnight and applied externally to sensitive areas.

White Pine: Tincture made from inner bark and needles applied externally only.

Diabetes

Grey Wolf believed stress and poor diet were the main causes.

Recommended Foods: Turmeric, grapefruit, broccoli, garlic, walnuts, and dandelion tea.

— Eliminate chemically refined sugars. Use organic raw coconut palm sugar sparingly as an alternative.
— Lifestyle: Focus on exercise, pure water, and fresh air.

Shingles
Often a sign of a weakened immune system.
Helpful Foods (Lysine): Fish, yogurt, apples, pears, and asparagus.
Avoid (Arginine): Tomatoes, nuts, chocolate, and sugars while active.
Relief: A wash cloth soaked in apple cider vinegar applied to the sores provides relief and helps them dry.

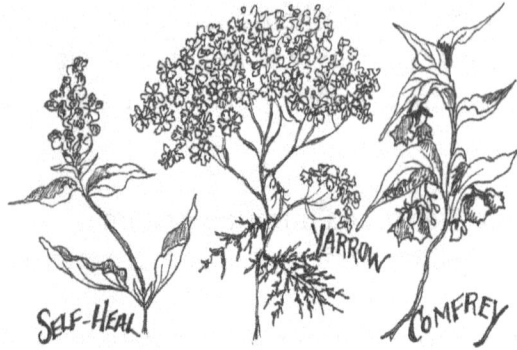

The Power Of Plants

Now I would like to talk about plants. If you took the time to notice their functions, you would soon find that plants send off a sense of well-being—a feeling of contentment, so to speak. They can enhance the appreciation of a moment or help a person deal with stress.

Old Grey Wolf said that some plants could correct multiple kinds of pain, reduce inflammation throughout the body, and relax muscles just by being in the house. Today I believe that millions of people lose their quality of life to chronic pain. Truth be known, some of these problems could be eliminated by seeking out what Mother Nature has to offer. It bothers me to no end to see folks suffering when the cure is usually only a few feet from their front door.

I would also like to mention a theory my Grandfather told me. He believed, as I do today, that if one dwells on the word pain, they will have pain. If a person continues to focus on it, it will get worse instead of better. The only way pain is eliminated is by focusing on other things. Happy thoughts.

Now comes an exciting fact of life. For many years I have ventured into how the mind works. Most would think this is impossible, but it isn't really; it is just looking beyond the realm of reality. I have found that the tastes and smells from plants have a wide-ranging influence on mental function.

Where certain things are absent in the brain, the smells and tastes from plants can protect brain cells from over-excitement, which contributes to the damaging effects of stroke, epilepsy, and other disorders.

It seems today folks want a magic pill without doing any of the work. They don't want to make changes in their life to correct the problem. They want to go to the doctor, get a pill, and come home hoping all their problems go away without changing one thing in their daily routine. It doesn't happen that way; it really doesn't.

I have often scratched my head while pondering how a person can go to a doctor's office and, within fifteen minutes, come out with a solution to a problem that has plagued them for months or years. My friend Grey Wolf told me years ago—and he lived to be 101—that he would sometimes spend days with folks figuring out what was wrong. He would live with them and watch their daily routine. Only then would he put together a plan.

Today we have X-rays, biopsies, and blood tests. Are all these tests good for you? From my own experience, I believe many of these procedures were unnecessary for me. I have had things done that caused me to suffer repeatedly for over thirty years. I would turn back the clock if I could. That is one reason I am writing this book; I hope to prevent others from going through unnecessary agony.

I believe the body can heal itself in most cases. If you find your body is failing you, take a very close look at your lifestyle. No magic pill will cure these problems permanently. Take an inventory. Go to the fridge and cupboards. Throw out the processed foods, most dairy (except a bit of aged cheese), and most meats. Chemical-free or wild game is good. Discard farm-grown fish; freshly caught is better. Remove white sugar and replace it with organic coconut palm sugar. Get rid of vegetable oils and lard, replacing them with coconut oil, cold-pressed olive oil, or real organic butter.

Then do the same with your thinking. Clean it up. Remove the stress. Grey Wolf said many times that a person usually becomes their own problem. Next, look at your laundry soaps. Replace them with natural, organic substances. Throw out fabric softeners—they are full of chemicals and scents that wreak havoc on the mind and sinuses. Use vinegar instead, mixed half-and-half with clean water. For shampoos and hand soap, use organic versions. To wash your hair, you can use baking soda.

To wash: Hold a half-pint of baking soda up to the shower nozzle. Let just enough water in to create a mixture. Work it into the hair and scalp, then rinse. To rinse: Pour a couple of ounces of organic apple cider vinegar over your hair, work it in, and rinse clean. It clears the mind and leaves the hair looking great.

Once you put this new lifestyle into motion, you will feel better mentally because you know you are doing what is right. Your thinking will become more evident. Most health-related problems would cease to exist quite quickly by putting this formula into action.

My Grandfather used to say that no changes can be forced upon a person. They have to want it, then be ready for it when it happens.

Other Items Of Interest

My Grandmothers Cranberry Sauce:

1-1/2 cups sugar (revised with raw organic coconut palm
sugar)
1 navel orange
1/2 tsp grated ginger
4 cups cranberries
1/2 cup (2 oz.) toasted pecans
Grate the orange peel and add to a pot with the sugar and
ginger. Add the juice from the orange into the pot and simmer
over medium heat until the sugar is dissolved. Add cranberries
and cook until they pop—about 5 minutes. Add pecans and
cool sauce.

Sweet Potatoes Stuffed with Cranberries:
1-1/2 cups of cranberry sauce
3 tbs butter
1/3 cup coconut palm sugar
1 tsp salt

1/2 cup chopped nuts

Bake potatoes until tender and easily peelable, about 30 minutes. Peel the skins, cut in half lengthwise. Scoop out some insides and reserve. Mash and stuff both halves holding the potato back together with toothpicks. Place in a greased oven pan. Mix sauce, nuts, sugar, butter, salt and pour over. Bake at 350 uncovered until lightly browned, about 20-25 minutes. It goes well with turkey, roast chicken, or duck. For less work don't hollow and stuff the potatoes, chunk them and pour sauce over them. Pretty tasty and so good for you.

Red Clover Tea:

Part used: Flower. Red clover is believed to combat cancer from forming and can also be used as a blood cleanser. The whole plant, infusion, or oil is used to treat many health complaints, ranging from coughs and fevers to high cholesterol and fertility problems. It is also capable of relaxing spasms and will help release water retention and induce sweating when needed. Its red flower lets one know about its blood-cleansing capabilities. Place 1 tbs of fresh or dried red clover blossoms in a cup. Pour 1-1/2 cup boiling water over the blossoms and let sit for five minutes. Add sweetener if desired. Tastes great.

Potassium Gluconate:

My sources say that potassium can help a lot of folks with back pain, joints, deteriorated discs, stiffness in arms, legs, fingers, neck, shoulders and many more problems. Potassium is about the best-kept secret in the reduction of pain that can occur throughout one's body. Grey Wolf used it to treat folks for years saying there is no better. All the problems above can be helped considerably by taking a 1/2 pill a day to start things off. See how your stomach reacts before increasing the amount. The results will astound you. I had it brought to my attention by a lady chiropractor in Florida. Great lady. She told me that for spasms in my lower back, that if I would take one half, 595 mg tablets when problems arise I would be walking within a couple of hours. She was right. I have them on hand all the time and never go anywhere without them. I would also like to mention here that I believe that a good chiropractor can be an asset to one's health. I feel what is needed is a chiropractor that will talk to you, assess your problem and then adjust your problem physically. Like putting joints and things back into place.

The trick, of course, is to find a good one. They are out there; we just have to ask around; find out how they treat their patients and then act accordingly. Worth mentioning that you can make potassium. Using organic vegetables, fill a large pot with 25 percent potato peelings, 25 percent carrot and beet peelings, 25 percent chopped onions and garlic, and 25 percent celery and greens. Add minced fresh chilies, such as jalapenos or crushed red pepper flakes to taste or more cooling herbs like thyme and marjoram. Add enough good water to cover the vegetables and simmer over a very low temperature for an hour. Now you strain. This will keep your body more alkaline which is a good thing and is also very useful for acidic conditions like arthritis or gout.

If you do opt to buy potassium over the counter remember this. Don't go and buy the most expensive product there is, as potassium is potassium, it is all pretty much the same. I should mention here though that if you are on heart medicine or have heart problems ask your doctor before taking potassium. Potassium works by relaxing your muscles and nerves; your heart is a muscle. Also, pregnant women should not take potassium without asking their health care provider.

Liver Aid:
   1 cup organic apple juice
   2 or 3 lemons freshly squeezed juice
   1 cup fresh water, distilled water, or filtered water
   1 clove fresh garlic

1 tablespoon virgin olive oil

1/4 inch fresh ginger-root

Lemon juice becomes alkaline in the stomach, which is an aid to the cleansing of the digestive tract; it will also help dissolve the olive oil. If you are unable to digest any citrus, use a teaspoon of turmeric instead. The garlic is best crushed before it is put into the blender. Blend all the ingredients until they form a smooth liquid. Pour into a glass or cup and drink it slowly. No more than a half a cup a day, for two days. Best taken in the morning instead of having breakfast. Then have a good lunch. Grey Wolf notes said he used milk-thistle for all types of liver troubles. It is available in most health-food stores. It also grows wild pretty well all over North American which would be my choice.

Water Retention:

If you have water retention problems, sprinkle plenty of celery seeds on your food. Or drink a 1 cup of dandelion root tea for three days. You can use dried or fresh. If in season, dig the root from dandelion, grind and put into a tea ball and let soak in a cup of hot water that has been previously boiled for five minutes. Then drink.

Pink Eye:

Pink Eye can be itchy, painful and red, usually caused by infections. There is also a viral and bacterial type pink eye caused by touching something with the virus or bacteria and rubbing the eyes. Smoke also will take its toll on the eyes, be it from cigarettes or stoking a fire. So what is one to do?

Once you are sure it is pink eye, you can now treat the condition using a natural remedy readily available to anyone. 1 teaspoon of dried chamomile (a tea bag is fine, loose is better), 1 teaspoonful of dried raspberry leaves, 5-6 petals off a wild rose (or 1 teaspoonful of dried grape root). Once you have your tea made you can use an eyedropper to wash your eyes. I use an eye-cup that can be purchased at any health food store. Make sure you strain your mixture well before putting into your eyes. Never use the same solution that you used in your infected eye in your good eye, doing so will infect it as well.

One last thing. The best preventative way of stopping most all eye problems, colds and flu's, is not to touch your eyes with unwashed hands.

Calendula:

The Calendula can help immensely with the prevention of muscle spasms, and it also helps to lower fevers if necessary. Grey Wolf used the petals to treat those suffering from a sore throat. Make into a tea and gargle with it three times a day. Very good for healing sores in the mouth. He goes on to say in his notes that a tea made from the petals, drank twice a day would be a great help for those that have cancer or a duodenal ulcer. It helped me a lot. This is how you make it. Put 1 to 2 teaspoons of dried flowers into 1 cup of hot water and let sit for 10 minutes. Strain and drink. Two cups a day if you like. My Grandmother said you could also use it externally for treating varicose veins, and hemorrhoids. Make into a tea and use as a wash when needed. They are easily grown and come back year after year all on their own. Birds love them along with the bees. A great asset to have planted in among your gardens. When in flower remove petals, dry and store in sealed mason jars for future use. Mark the jars with dates and discard after two years.

Apple Tree Bark:

Some have used the bark to create a tonic that will treat gravel in the bladder and also aid in reducing fever naturally if needed.

Alfalfa:

A highly nutritious herb, good for the mind, it also alkalizes the body rapidly and detoxifies the liver. I also found it helps a lot in rebuilding decayed teeth and helps those with arthritis and rheumatic pain.

Aloe Vera: Aloe Vera is good for burns. While this is well known, what you may not know is that aloe plants are also helpful in treating cancer and stomach ailments.

Balsam Poplar:
   Poplar buds, bark and leaves are used to alleviate the discomfort of cough colds, lung trouble and kidneys. The buds can also be used as a tea for gargling, making it an excellent remedy for sore throats, coughs and laryngitis.

Bee Pollen:
   Great for allergies and helps boost up the bodies immune system. It also helps those with radiation sickness, the kind people get when they undergo radiation therapy for cancer. If you so choose to take that route. If you do, make sure you do the research beforehand.

Kelp:
   Kelp is worth mentioning here in this book. Reason being that Grey Wolf used it to treat many different health-related issues. Taken from his notes, it is said it was excellent for problems of the thyroid gland and goitres. It also is very good for bringing the sensory nerves back to what they should be. Along with that it is very good for nails, hair and cleanses radiation from the body if one becomes exposed. Kind of think in today's world it would be a great added item to have in your medicine chest.

Papaya:

Papaya is a definite help for those having problems with digestion. It is also very useful in relieving allergies by its ability to break down proteins. I have used it as an enzyme for the relief of heartburn and the digestion of food with excellent results.

Sarsaparilla Root:

Sarsaparilla Root is used to eliminate poisons from the blood and purifies the system from infections. It can also be used to treat rheumatism, gout, skin eruptions, ringworm, internal inflammation and colds. Not the easiest to find, so when you do, stock up on it as it lasts for years if stored in sealed jars. Grey Wolf said that in the American "Old West," sarsaparilla was the most popular drink of the cowboys. I have to agree, as I drank it quite a few times growing up and nothing was more enjoyable.

White Oak Bark:

The bark here in Canada and most parts of the USA is readily available. It is excellent for treating varicose veins. My Grandfather said it was about the best remedy out there for piles and hemorrhoids or any trouble of the rectum. Found in most health stores, or if you have a white oak tree on your property or nearby harvest your own. Simple to do, just peel of some bark from the smaller branches and dry. Grind and use when needed. Make a tea solution, then applied to affected areas, 1 tbs per cup of hot water.

Carrots:

Grey Wolf swore that carrots could fix just about anything. Here are some healing properties that they give us. Benefits the Lungs, is an anti-inflammatory for mucous membranes, eases whooping cough and reduces coughs in general. Strengthens the spleen and pancreas. Improves liver function. Stimulates the elimination of wastes. Helps dissolve kidney and gallbladder stones. Helps dissolve tumours that aren't necessary for the body to stay healthy. Benefits the stomach by reducing excess stomach acid, good for heartburn and acid reflux. Eliminates dangerous bacteria in the intestines and good for diarrhea. Benefits the eyes & improves vision. Great for skin irritations and heals burns when the juice is applied directly to the skin. Increases mother's milk for breastfeeding. They even destroy intestinal parasites like pinworms and roundworms. Benefits the ears, improves hearing and clears up earaches.

Red Clover:
Red clover is an excellent blood purifier. It is said that it helps eliminate most forms of cancer, containing lime, silica and other earthy salts. It also causes a relaxing sensation to nerves and the entire system. White clover works about as well as red clover and is found anywhere in North America.

Rose Hips:
Rose Hips contains a great deal of vitamin C, ranging from 10 to 100 times greater than any other known food. Knowing this it can be used as an infection fighter. It can also help with physical stress and pollution of the body. A few more vitamins that it contains is, A, B1, B2, E, K, P, niacin, calcium, iron and phosphorous. Soon as the flowers start to fall one should keep an eye open for the rose hips, they look like a small red cherry but much harder. My wife and I gather them, dry them and store in sealed mason jars, to be crushed when needed for teas. Great tasting too and so good for you.

Stinging Nettle:
Stinging Nettle is readily available throughout North America. They are found all over the world. Grey Wolf said that the smallest amount would strengthen the entire body within days. He also said it was very helpful for those dealing

with rheumatism, arthritis, eczema, nosebleeds, cleansing of the arteries and also helps in lowering one's blood pressure. Edible parts are leaves, stems and roots. Young leaves are preferable, however, no matter how far into the growing season be sure to remember that until dried or cooked, stinging nettle leaves will have those stinging hairs. (Never eat them raw!) Nettles make an excellent spinach substitute and can be added to soups and stews. Nettle root is excellent for an enlarged prostate when urination is painful. A tea made from the leaves is rich in iron and is an excellent detoxifier for the body. Nettles contain calcium, chlorine, iron, potassium, silicon, sodium and sulphur, all tremendous nutritional factors.

Caution: When collecting stinging nettle always cover up all exposed skin. The swollen base of each tiny hollow hair contains a droplet of formic acid. When the hair tip pierces the skin, the acid makes it into the skin causing an annoying itch or burning that can last several minutes up to a couple of days. Grey wolf said that by rubbing the stings with stinging nettle root or jewel-weed, has been used to suppress the itch/burning sensation. It seems to me that Mother Nature has its problems now and again, but not too far away is the fix. It is a much-overlooked herb that in my opinion should be called upon more often.

Mallow Root:
Mallow Root is excellent to bathe sore and inflamed eyes when made into a tea. Next, to raspberry leaves, there is none better. It also is quite good for lung problems, hoarseness, diarrhea and all kidney diseases. Great to have on hand.

Licorice:
Licorice contains natural cortisone. Grey Wolf said it had been used for years to treat ailments of the glands and stress. It is also quite good for coughs and chest problems due to colds or difficulties breathing. It is quite useful in the treatment of

gastric ulcers and throat conditions. My wife and I have used it for years for all kinds of different ailments with excellent results. Seek out natural licorice, not the ladened sugar types bought on the candy shelves.

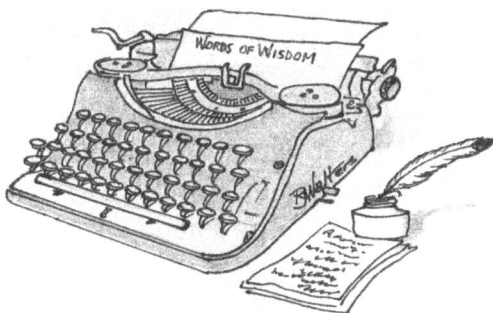

Words Of Wisdom

Now nearing the end of this book, I would like to share a few words of wisdom that came to me through visions, family and friends. Enjoy!

To be half Native is to take the best of both worlds and reject what's left. Most folks are continually waiting for life to begin. Myself I never waited. I live each day.

The fact is, we have been programmed right from birth. Right from the day we are born children are told what to do. The adult chooses their name, what religion they will follow, or God they will worship, what education they will need, what clothes they should wear and much more. Is this wrong? Well in some respects I believe it is.

I believe we have to reprogram ourselves if we want to find our real purpose in life. We all have a purpose and a road to follow, just nowadays most don't. It's never too late though, and if asked I would suggest, you get on with it.

1 — Burn sage and cedar, then ask questions. The smoke brings on good luck and wards off evil spirits and things. Grandmother earth will refuse to hide evil spirits. The smoke will reveal everything to you so be prepared.

2 — There is more within Nature than a person can see with their eyes, more than they can ever hope to understand.

3 — People today have the feeling that what is different may expose them to danger. That's the reason they shy away from Natures medicines and way of life.

4 — I believe in leaving Nature alone and trying to learn from her, instead of trying to master her.

5 — When you work with the soil day in and day out, it gives you respect for life.

6 — The trick is you have to remember there are all kinds of plants that will kill you deader than a door-nail if you eat them raw. But cook them up, and they are lip-smacking good, and some will kill you, raw or cooked. You have got to learn to live with it. Education!

7 — I've lived with fear long enough now not to be shoved around by it, foolishly.

8 — Fear is like a fire in dry grass. It spreads easily.

9 — See yourself as you want to be. See it, feel it, hear it, believe it, make it real.

10 — Breath in filling lungs with everything healthy. Breath out releasing everything bad.

11 — Talk out loud to your cells, blood, skin cells, all cells to seek out the problems and eliminate it.

12 — Why does everything in life change? I don't know the answer to that. I only know it does, and that you can't stop it. What you can do is figure how to deal with it.

13 — Sometimes a person has to swallow hard and accept what he could not change.

14 — Only after the last tree has been cut down, only after the last river has been poisoned, only after the last fish has been caught—then will you find that money cannot be eaten. "Cree Prophecy"

15 — Some things have short life's compared to ours, like tulips. Trees now, on the other hand, have long life's, some over two hundred years of age.

16 — I have found that I was redefined by natures offerings during my wanderings through her treasures. It's hard now to deny my own existence and truth be known, I don't want to be at any other time than now.

17 — Myself I believe that all things in Nature are connected, humans included and that forms of spirituality can promote health, or cause illness. Therefore, it is necessary to heal not only the physical parts of an individual, but also their emotional wellness, and their harmony with what and who lives around them. Do this, and it is my feeling the world would be a lot better off.

18 — Some folks say beauty can only be seen, but I say, that is wrong. Beauty is where you are at in life at that moment, around, beside or in one's self, one just has to let his or her mind do whatever it chooses.

19 — Each person is responsible for their health, and all thoughts and actions have consequences, including illness, disability, bad luck, or trauma. Only when harmony is set right, can your health be restored.

20 — Remember, we all can heal ourselves – we don't need toxic drugs to get healthy.

21 — The best doctor in the world is you. Your health is your responsibility, take it back. We should be educating not medicating. You have to open your eyes. You have to do it yourself. You have to walk the walk.

22 — Your body is fantastic, it just needs to be healthy. It wants to be healthy.

23 — Think about the positive, happy people you know. If you can count more than five, it's a sign that you are one of them. Because positive people like to be among positive people!

24 — If we are wounded, we go to our mother and seek to lay the injured part against her, to be healed. Animals do too; they put their wounds to the earth.

25 — Harvest only what you can use yourself. Please respect every plant's right to survive and reproduce. Be informed as to the effects your harvesting will have on the survival of the plant, and the surrounding environment.

26 — The Great Spirit is our father, but the earth is our mother. She nourishes us, and what we put into the ground she returns to us, and healing plants she gives to us.

If you take the time to talk to Nature you will begin to know each other. If you don't talk to Nature you will not know her and what we don't know we fear. What we fear we then destroy.

Poem

GREY WOLF'S CURE

One day as Reg and George were talking
After the farm chores at their home were all done;
Let's go visit our old friend Jim, said Reg,
It'll be a nice ride in the warm morning sun!

So away they went with the horse and the buggy
And arrived in about an hour or so;
Old Jim, it seemed, had a touch of the rheumatism
And was walking kind of careful and slow!

Well, they visited with Jim for a couple of hours
And then headed back home to the farm;
Laura would have a nice supper all ready
And the horse would go back to the barn!

So later on that very next day,
As to Reg and Laura George was talking;
I think I'll go and visit my old friend Grey Wolf,
For it is a beautiful day for walking!

Grey Wolf lived not very far away,
In a little cabin, down by the creek;
Maybe he could help their neighbour Jim,
So with Grey Wolf, George was eager to speak!

Grey Wolf was sitting on his front porch,
Whittling a piece of ash;

It helped him with his meditation

And it didn't cost him any cash!

Grey Wolf was George's best friend,
From so many years ago;
He taught George about the ways of Mother Nature
In the spring, summer, fall and the snow!
So Grey Wolf said he had an old remedy,
That was passed on from years ago;
He said,'We'll make a potion for Jim',
'He'll feel better in a few days or so'!

He gathered some leaves from an old cedar tree
And to 'The Great Spirit' Grey Wolf gave his thanks;
He promised to reward the tree with two fishes,
That he would soon catch down by the river bank!

So they ground up the leaves in an old wooden bowl
And on the stove they warmed up some lard;
Then they added in some comfrey roots,
From outside the cabin in the yard!

They mixed everything together,
About a handful of each ingredient was needed;
Then they strained the potion through a clean white cloth,
Before the afternoon sun had receded!

So George gave the potion to his old friend Jim,
With instructions on how to use it;
In a couple of weeks Jim was feeling just fine
And was walking around good and fit!

So Jim said to give Grey Wolf his thanks,
For his handed-down home-made potion;

'And tell him to drop in for supper sometime',
'If he ever happens to get the notion'!

So there you have it, a home-made remedy,
Tried and true and it works just fine;
Thanks to George's old friend Grey Wolf
And Mother Nature's trees, plants and sunshine!

So if you happen to have some ailments
And your wits are at their end;
Pay close attention to **Mother Nature's** bounty,
She will be forever your best friend!

By Bob Bartlett

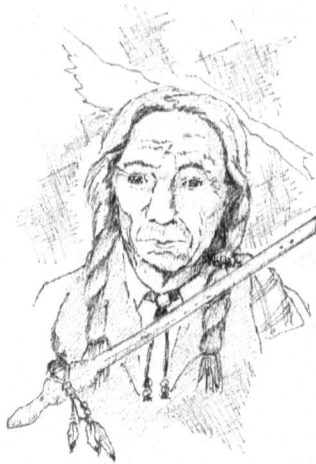

Grey Wolf's Words

While sitting one day, Grey Wolf got to talking about people in general. He said. "You know, I read an excellent article awhile back which said that we are very careless people in many ways. We travel at a furious pace and couldn't care less about the results."

It goes on to say that a great many ills and diseases can be avoided. Take a person that is very warm, thirsty and sweating. How many in this condition will pour ice water into their stomachs producing gastritis, which is inflammation of the stomach? Or, perhaps bring on a severe chill from doing so.

How many now sit down in this condition in a draft causing one to catch a cold, sore throat, pneumonia, bronchitis, or bring on pain of rheumatism? How many will get their clothes or their shoes and stockings wet and sit in them for hours on end and then wonder why they feel sick?

How many will work or dance themselves into perspiration and then sit in a cool place to cool off quickly and wonder why they have coughs, headaches, and feel sickly all over. (Nasal problems, chronic sore throat, laryngitis and consumption flourish on such mistakes.)

How many people will drink the most potent kinds of teas and coffees, live on them so to speak for breakfast, and then wonder why their stomach and nerves are sick, or their bowels are constipated and livers sluggish? How many will continually eat ham, pork, sausage, rich pies and cakes, greasy gravies, warm pancakes and then top things off with tea or coffee or wines and liqueurs; and then continue living an unaroused life and wonder why their stomachs give out, and they have indigestion, nauseousness or feel like they are wasting away? You cannot disobey the laws of Nature or health and remain well my friends.

I have seen parents give a ten-year-old baby rich cookies, candies and maple syrup and even peanuts and wonder why the baby cry's with a sore stomach, rushing the child off to a doctor. I have seen parents give their children green apples or overripe bananas which again put them in the hospital or doctor's office wondering what is wrong. We reap what we sow, whether we sow it intentionally or otherwise.

How can you escape from rheumatism if you live in a cold, damp, musty house which is closed against sunlight? You can't. All these instances above could be prevented and remember, preventive treatment is the only sure treatment. Treat yourself and your children how to eat, drink and act, and how to live, it's the only way to be healthy both physically and morally.

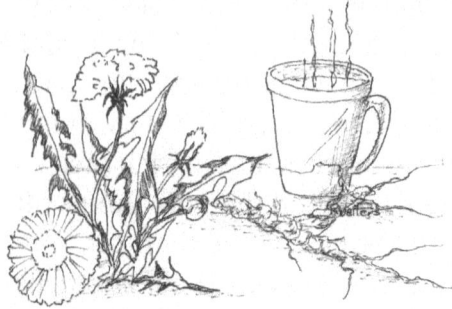

The Dandelion

Now, at the end of this book, a few words about a plant that is a powerful ally for health. Over the years I have done major research on the dandelion. I have found that it not only makes certain harmful cells self-destruct without hurting the good cells, it also builds up the immune system which then can fight off many future problems and ailments.

The research suggests it works well against many serious conditions. It takes time and one has to learn patience. I like to dig the dandelion in season, roots, leaves and flower. Making sure that the soil where I was digging was free of all chemicals and not so good things.

I then bring one whole plant into the house where my wife washes it, grinds it up and puts it in a pot with about two cups of water and simmers it. She makes sure that the water isn't boiling as that would remove all the good properties. Stirring occasionally. Once finished she strains it into cups and we drink it. Pretty tasty by itself. Today we both drink dandelion tea once in a while as in doing so keeps the body in a healthy state.

This is how I, in part, believe the body can be brought back to health. I start digging them as soon as they come out in the spring. I dig a bunch of them, mostly the roots. By taking a shovel shoving it down beside them and move it around to loosen the soil. I then reach down, get a firm grip on the top of the root and pull it out very slowly. Most of the time they will break, which is okay, as it will grow again for next year.

Once gathered, I take them in the house, cut them up and dry them. I don't take the soil off, I leave it on. After the soil is dry I remove most of the soil leaving a wee bit. I learned it was a vital part in helping the body get better. Now I make sure they are dry to where they snap. I dry mine in my oven as it is propane and has a pilot light, which dries them perfectly. The key here is not to heat them up above 104 degrees F, as that would kill all the good nutrients.

I also hang them like you would onions from a high place where the air can circulate around them. Once dry I take the whole root, break it in half and put them in mason jars for winter. I needed around three quarts to last me through winter. Then when needed I would take a cup full, grind them up with a mortar and pestle. The soil that is left on the roots plays a major role in the healing process, one teaspoon a day in a glass of cold water.

I took this until my stomach felt a bit acidic or nauseous. For me it was six months, then I cut back to a half a teaspoon and kept cutting back till I was down to nothing. I had to learn what my body needed; I accomplished this by paying attention to my body. Once I got to this point I believed my health was restored. Now my body was built back to where it should be. It has worked well for me along with others; I am sure it could be of help to anyone else.

If Nature could only speak to us, she'd say. "This is what this contains, and you need it." I also keep tabs on my pH these days with strips. There is no better way to find out where your body is at. Most folks that have serious illness if checked would find their body is very acidic. Mine was about five when I started. I changed my lifestyle, today it sets around 7.0 to 7.4. Occasionally I bring it up to around 8 just to make sure things are as they should be.

It does take time, and one has to learn patience. Illness loves a low pH, thrives in it. We, like our soil, should also be about 7 to 7.5. I check my urine first thing in the morning, which usually reads 6.5 or a bit higher. Where it should be. I also check it before eating or drinking anything. One last thing about the soil being left on the roots. I have come to believe that the soil has a type of bacteria in it, and if taken internally can bring damaged cells back to a healthy normal cell.

Make sure the soil is free of dangerous chemicals.

While writing this book, (in the news) I see they have found a new antibiotic which comes from soil bacteria. Pretty amazing. Just reassures me that I am right in my thinking.

My wife Ruth and I wish you great success in your future endeavours, using:

Nature's Gateway To Health.

Thank You for Reading

If you enjoyed this book, all of my titles are available on Amazon. I would truly appreciate hearing your thoughts.

Leaving a short review or comment helps other readers discover my work, and every one of them means a great deal to me.

Thank you for taking the time to read.

George Walters

www.ingramcontent.com/pod-product-compliance
Lightning Source LLC
Chambersburg PA
CBHW071346290326
41933CB00041B/2731